William A. Haseltine

ANNA DIRKSEN

Voices in Dementia Care

Reimagining the Culture of Care

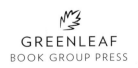

GREENLEAF
BOOK GROUP PRESS

This book is intended as a reference volume only, not as a medical manual. The information given here is designed to help you make informed decisions about your health. It is not intended as a substitute for any treatment that may have been prescribed by your doctor. If you suspect that you have a medical problem, you should seek competent medical help. You should not begin a new health regimen without first consulting a medical professional.

Published by Greenleaf Book Group Press
Austin, Texas
www.gbgpress.com

Copyright ©2018 ACCESS Health International

All rights reserved.

Previously published by Tethys, an imprint of Yatra Books, 2018, India, 978-93-83125-16-6

Distributed by Greenleaf Book Group

For ordering information or special discounts for bulk purchases, please contact Greenleaf Book Group at PO Box 91869, Austin, TX 78709, 512.891.6100.

Design and composition by Greenleaf Book Group
Cover design by Greenleaf Book Group

Publisher's Cataloging-in-Publication data is available.

Print ISBN: 978-1-62634-693-2

eBook ISBN: 978-1-62634-694-9

Part of the Tree Neutral® program, which offsets the number of trees consumed in the production and printing of this book by taking proactive steps, such as planting trees in direct proportion to the number of trees used: www.treeneutral.com

TreeNeutral

Printed in the United States of America on acid-free paper

19 20 21 22 23 24 25   10 9 8 7 6 5 4 3 2 1

Second Edition

All people, no matter where they live, no matter what their age, have the right to access high quality and affordable healthcare and to lead healthy and productive lives.

Acknowledgments

Voices in Dementia Care is based on a series of interviews with dementia care experts across Europe and the United States. The authors of this book are deeply grateful to all those who took the time to sit with us and share their insight and expertise on dementia care. We have been inspired by your passion for the work and are humbled to be allowed to share that passion with a wider audience.

We are equally grateful to our ACCESS Health colleagues, Jean Galiana and Sofia Widén, for researching and conducting the interviews and for the time they took to carefully review and edit the final transcripts.

Gary Weber was an early and constant supporter of ACCESS Health work on elder, long-term, and dementia care in Sweden. The William A. Haseltine Foundation provided funding and support for the work in both the United States and Sweden. We are grateful to both of our funders.

Contents

Innovative Approaches to Dementia Care

DEMENTIA takes a toll on every person it touches: the person living with dementia and their loved ones, caregivers, family, and friends. There is no telling when or whom it will strike. The most common type of dementia, Alzheimer's disease, destroys both physical and cognitive skills. Eventually, it prevents a person from carrying out even the simplest of tasks.

People living with Alzheimer's often liken it to a fog that rolls in, preventing a person from making sense of the world around them. Brian LeBlanc is a national public speaker and an advocate for dementia awareness and education. Four generations of his family have been diagnosed with Alzheimer's disease. In October of 2014, he was diagnosed as well. Still in the early stages, Mr. LeBlanc describes his experience with the disease in his blog A Little Bit of Brilliance.[1]

---

1   LeBlanc, B. (2015, March 14). Fog: It's Not Just a Weather Condition. Retrieved October 13, 2017, from https://abitofbriansbrilliance.com/2015/03/14/fog-its-not-just-a-weather-condition/

[I]magine driving down the road. Fog has set in and visibility is obstructed. You can't see much, you're cautious of your surroundings because of the dense fog. All of a sudden, you break through to a clearing. You can see all around you…

You get up to get something, the fog rolls in, preventing you from remembering where you are or why you're there. You're in the middle of a conversation, the fog rolls in so thick it turns to night, blocking out every thought, rendering you speechless. You're driving to a very familiar place, again the fog rolls in and you have no idea where you are. You have to rely on your GPS to tell you where to go.

This isn't just sporadic or a one-time event. This is every day, several times a day, a typical day. Sometimes the fog is thicker, sometimes less, but it's ALWAYS there. It's my Alzheimer's journey.

Other common forms of dementia, such as vascular dementia, Lewy body dementia, and frontotemporal disorders, can be equally gruelling for both individuals and the people who care for them. Yet, while the toll dementia takes on an individual and their family is immense, the toll it is taking on societies as a whole is even greater.

The Global Impact of Dementia

Nearly fifty million people globally are living with dementia. The condition strikes so often and so arbitrarily that is has been dubbed "The Silent Epidemic." The number of people with dementia is expected to double every twenty years, reaching seventy-five million in 2030 and 131.5 million in 2050.[2]

The greatest increases are occurring in low and middle income countries. Already, more than half of all people with

---

2   Prince, M., Comas-Herrera, A., Knapp, M., Guerchet, M., & Karagiannidou, M. (2016). World Alzheimer Report 2016: Improving healthcare for people living with dementia. *Alzheimers & Dementia*. doi:10.1016/j.jalz.2015.06.1858

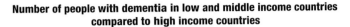

Number of people with dementia in low and middle income countries compared to high income countries

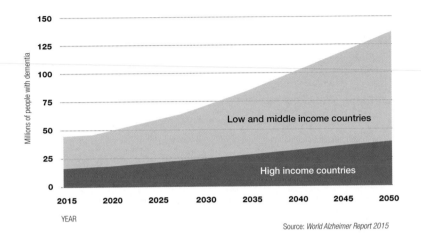

Source: *World Alzheimer Report 2015*

dementia live in low and middle income countries. By 2050, that number will rise to more than two-thirds. When looking at total deaths due to dementia, China and India are at the top of the list, due to the sheer size of their populations and despite the fact that dementias actually make up a small proportion of total deaths. When adjusted for differences in population size, the country with the highest number of deaths due to dementia is actually Finland.[3]

Much of the increase in dementia rates and deaths due to dementia is fueled by demographic change, with people in rich and poor countries alike living longer lives. The number of people over the age of sixty is expected to more than double by 2050 and more than triple by 2100. While dementia is not caused by aging, it is much more prevalent among older individuals compared to the young. At present, the global population of people sixty and older is growing faster than any other age group.

---

3 VanderZanden, A. (2014, December). A closer look at Alzheimer's disease worldwide. Retrieved October 13, 2017, from http://www.healthdata.org/newsletters/impact-13/deep-dive

Across the board, countries and communities must begin to bear an increasingly heavy burden of costs for dementia care and treatment. Dementia is a complicated disorder and providing high quality, coordinated, and low cost care is a challenge for any country. In low and middle income settings, where healthcare resources are already stretched thin, the challenge is even more daunting.

Many recent studies have shown that significant improvements are needed in the diagnosis and treatment of dementia, especially in terms of access to services, disease management, and communication and coordination.[4] People with dementia often receive fragmented and uncoordinated care that does not properly address their needs or the needs of the friends and family who care for them. Even the initial step to treatment—diagnosis—is out of reach for most. The vast majority of individuals with dementia have never been diagnosed.

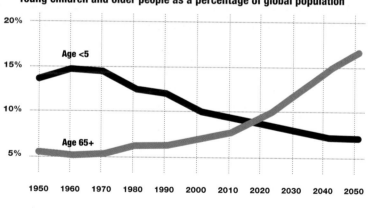

Young children and older people as a percentage of global population

Source: United Nations. *World Population Prospects: The 2010 Revision.*
Available at: http://esa.un.org/undp/wpp

---

4   Prorok, J. C., Horgan, S., & Seitz, D. P. (2013). Health care experiences of people with dementia and their caregivers: a meta-ethnographic analysis of qualitative studies. *Canadian Medical Association Journal*, 185(14). doi:10.1503/cmaj.121795

ACCESS Health International is a global nonprofit committed to ensuring that all people, no matter what their age or health condition, have access to high quality and affordable care. Over the past two years, Jean Galiana and Sofia Widén of ACCESS Health have interviewed more than sixty pioneers in elder care and dementia care in Denmark, Norway, the Netherlands, and across the United States. These interviews have helped us identify best practices in dementia care. Our analysis of these practices can help public and private healthcare providers implement new and more cost effective ways to deliver care. They can also help individuals living with dementia and their caregivers understand innovative options for care that they may not know exist.

In the pages that follow this opening analysis, we include transcripts of our interviews with the elder care and long-term care providers we have interviewed about dementia care. The voices of these care professionals are important to hear in their entirety, as they describe the nuances of the challenges inherent in delivering innovative high quality dementia care with limited resources.

Based on our analysis of these interviews, we have identified the critical best practices that we believe all elder and long-term care providers should consider when delivering care to people living with dementia. These best practices can be adapted and applied by the informal caregiver as well—the sister, brother, child, or other loved one who may be responsible for caring for a person living with dementia outside of a traditional care environment.

The Importance of Inclusion

One overarching best practice that should be applied to each of the sections below is the concept of inclusion. This idea is best explained in our interview with the Dementia Action Alliance, a diverse coalition of activists working to create a better society for individuals who live with dementia. Karen Love is the Executive Director of the Alliance. She describes the catalyst for the creation of the Alliance, which was formed after she and other individuals passionate about dementia learned that the government had built a federal advisory council made up of researchers and clinicians but not a single person living with dementia.

She notes, "[The perspective of people living with dementia] is crucial. They offer insights and solve issues from their unique vantage point. What could be better? I do not know why every organization dealing with any aspect of dementia does not include those living with dementia. They are an invaluable resource."

Ms. Love goes on to describe the importance of inclusion at an even broader level:

> People living with dementia also need to be included in society. As their condition progresses, a person living with dementia loses the ability to self-initiate. That is often the reason why those living with dementia are not doing anything. They are inactive not because they do not want to be active, but because they need to be kick started through engagement. Inclusion and involvement is better for their health. It is better for their overall well-being. Many basic needs of people living with dementia, such as engagement, go unmet.

Love's colleague Jackie Pinkowitz, chair of the Alliance Board of Directors, described the concept of inclusion further:

> Karen and I were committed to the concept "nothing about us without us" from the very beginning of the Dementia Action

Alliance. The expression comes from the disability world. I used to teach special needs children, and later my mother developed Alzheimer's, so I had that philosophy and mindset. We knew that the voices of those living with dementia were not being heard anywhere that mattered. We created an advisory council entirely of people living with dementia.

The notion of inclusion applies to all best practices related to dementia care described below. Indeed, putting the person living with dementia at the center of the caregiving experience is among the most important best practices our research and analysis unearthed.

Person Centered Care

Person centered dementia care puts the person living with dementia at the center of all caregiving efforts and promotes quality of life regardless of physical or cognitive condition. This type of care honors a person's priorities, preferences, and personality, while still ensuring that their health and well-being are well taken care of.

Janne Rosvik is a registered nurse with a PhD in person centered care and dementia care from the University of Oslo. She has been working with the Norwegian Advisory Unit for Aging and Health for the past six years. Dr. Rosvik built on the work of two pioneers in dementia care, Tom Kitwood and Dawn Brooker, to develop a practical model of person centered caregiving based on four key elements: values, individuality, perspective, and social inclusion. This model has become known as the VIPS practice model.

In her interview with ACCESS Health, Dr. Rosvik describes a person centered model of care:

The core of person centered care is to think of a person with dementia as a person who has the same needs as everybody else. What is happening in his brain does not change his value as a person. It makes him a person with problems in the brain. His feelings and his emotions are still there, maybe even a bit stronger. When the person becomes agitated, which we often see, it may be because he is unable to express himself. We need to learn how to use all the knowledge we have about symptoms of dementia to try to understand the person's perspective on the world around him. What happens in his brain often makes it difficult for him to explain with words, so he may have to use other means of communication. It is our responsibility to learn his way of communicating. We don't just try to make this person nonaggressive; we try to understand him.

The VIPS practice model that Dr. Rosvik developed includes twenty-four indicators that guide caregivers in any situation, ensuring that they offer person centered care to the person living with dementia. The indicators are based on the four elements of the VIPS practice model, as Dr. Rosvik describes:

The "V" stands for the values of person centered care. The main value is that the person with dementia and the perspective of this person is just as important as our own perspectives as caregivers. The "I" is for individual care, which means we observe and note each person's unique traits. What is special about this person? What are his habits? What other illnesses does he have? The "P" is for perspective of the person. How does the world look from his point of view? The "S" is for social inclusion. Are his social needs taken care of? Is he included in social fellowship with other people? Each letter has six subindicators, which are used in the analysis that is part of the VIPS practice model. We check all twenty-four indicators and determine if any one of those is relevant to a given situation... Is the external environment here good for the person? Is there something in the environment that is disturbing him? Do we care about his perspective? Are his human rights taken care of? The "I," P," and "S" indicators are used most because they are more concrete, but we do not skip any of the four elements. This is how we make sure that person centered care is the focus.

This practical approach to implementing person centered care is echoed by Davina Porock, who was trained at the University of Bradford in person centered care and eventually established the University of Buffalo Institute for Person Centered Care in 2012. As part of her research with the Institute, she examined how to measure person centeredness and to determine that person centered care was actually occurring.

People used to say, "Oh, it is just about being nice. If everyone is just nice to the elderly people, we'll be fine." It is much more than that. Patient centeredness is not the classic picture of old people parked around the edge of the lounge room of the nursing home, asleep in their chairs. The practice of only keeping residents clean and dry actually does more harm than good.

People with more advanced dementia can have what are sometimes called "difficult behaviors." They can be aggressive. Sometimes they might hit, bite, or scream. People with advanced dementia can become agitated and pace the floor, trying to escape, or repeatedly call out. These behaviors are misunderstood.

Someone with dementia cannot comprehend what or who is coming at him or her. Someone with dementia cannot comprehend people talking or doing things quickly. The only thing they can do to take back control is to stop, hit, or resist in other ways. These behaviors need to be understood as stress reactions, not bad behavior. We have created a malignant social environment that does not treat these behaviors as distressed responses. Dementia patients have few other options than to respond negatively. Dementia patients want to have control over their environments and what happens to them, just like any other person.

We can reduce their stress by changing to a person centered approach. For example, we can change the way we speak to people. We can ensure that we do not take people by surprise. We can give visual cues such as hand cues to say what we are doing instead of only verbal cues. A specific example is to take the hand of the patient and help them clean their teeth rather than brushing their teeth for them. These changes are very simple things, but they all take time. People have to be reminded that these person centered approaches are important.

The challenge is how to apply the person centered care processes in institutional settings. It can be difficult to get traditional nursing homes to include the values, likes, and dislikes of the individual in their care model.

Applying Person Centered Care in a Long-Term Care Setting

While researchers like Dr. Rosvik and Ms. Porock consistently agree that person centered care is a best practice that must be applied to improve the quality of life and care for people living with dementia, ACCESS Health explored how that approach is actually delivered in nursing homes, elder care facilities, and other long-term care settings.

Lotta Roupe has worked as an elder care nurse in long-term care facilities for more than forty years. In 2001, she graduated from the one-year education program at Stiftelsen Silviahemmet, which is a nonprofit foundation dedicated to improving the quality of life for persons affected by dementia and their families. The cornerstones of the Silviahemmet philosophy include person centered care, along with team work, family support, communication, and relationship building. Ms. Roupe currently manages the Silviahemmet day care center in Stockholm, Sweden, which cares for young and elderly people affected by dementia.

Ms. Roupe describes how person centered care is realized daily at care facilities:

> If an individual starts looking for the bathroom and cannot find it, a staff member may intervene early to guide that person to the bathroom. This intervention prevents that person from feeling confused, anxious, or frustrated because he or she cannot find the bathroom.
>
> The role of caring for people who suffer from dementia involves knowing the person, being able to read signals, being able to step in and provide a hand of support, but also being able to reflect carefully upon when to intervene and when to step back . . .
>
> To deliver person centered dementia care, every caregiver needs to take the time to get to know the person who suffers from dementia. Caregivers need to create a relationship with the individual to deliver person centered care. Caregivers do this by spending time with the individual and talking about what matters to him or her. The caregivers eat together and sit down to have coffee with the visitors.

Ms. Roupe uses the term "visitors" to describe the people living with dementia who visit the day care center.

> The staff members are not viewed as caregivers, and they do not view themselves as caregivers. The staff members view themselves as friends of the visitors and they communicate in that way. This is an important element of the care philosophy,

especially for the younger elderly who suffer from dementia. The younger elderly do not want to be treated like patients. The younger elderly want to participate in activities and enjoy company during the day. The younger elderly need support but want to feel normal.

The staff members at the Silviahemmet day care center work closely together with the relatives of the visitors to ensure that every aspect of a visitor's needs is understood. Relatives receive a minimum of one update each month but are encouraged to be involved on a daily basis in what goes on at the day care center, either through visits, phone calls, text messages, or emails. Every six months, caregivers at the center reevaluate each person's care plan to make sure it is living up to the four cornerstones of the Silviahemmet philosophy. The care plan is constantly evaluated and revised to meet the needs of the visitors. Ms. Roupe shares an example of these kinds of revisions to the care plan:

> For example, one guest may be able to take long walks and paint in the beginning of his or her visits to the day care center. After about six months, the dementia may have caused certain physical and cognitive functions to deteriorate. That individual may no longer be able to paint or take long walks. That is why the staff members continuously update and revise the care plans. Every six months, we revise each component of the care philosophy to suit the individual and his or her needs. At the same time, we hold a continuous dialogue with the individual's relatives, since the relatives may also change their minds when the needs of the individual change.

Having staff members work together collaboratively to understand the needs of the people they care for is an approach also applied in the United States at the award winning dementia care center Vermilion Cliffs, located at the Beatitudes Campus retirement living and aging services center in Arizona. Staff members at Vermilion Cliffs meet weekly to discuss each resident and their individual needs and preferences. There is a fluid partnership with the families of residents—as is the case at Silviahemmet—to inform the design of the resident's care plan. The weekly meetings provide each member of the staff, from housekeepers all the way up to the directors of the center, with the knowledge needed to care for the residents and the autonomy to help them in any way they can.

Karen Mitchell is a registered nurse who has been working at Beatitudes Campus since 1983. She described how these weekly meetings have shaped the person centered and person directed care at Vermilion Cliffs:

> Everyone had to recognize that the needs and preferences of the residents were directing our policies and procedures. The residents are guiding us by how they respond to issues. Who knows the residents the best? The housekeeper who is in the room every day—not the management or the board.
>
> Our job as managers is to support the entire staff in doing what they know to be best for the residents. Everyone understands that culture.

Ms. Mitchell describes one incident that took place at Vermilion Cliffs while she was working as a nurse on one of the floors. One of the housekeepers noticed that a resident was not singing as she usually did in the morning. The next day, staff checked the temperature of the resident and noticed it was elevated. "[The resident] spiked a temperature due to a urinary tract infection," explained Ms.

Mitchell. "The housekeeper, who listened to the resident singing each day, detected the early sign of discomfort. She knew the resident well. Importantly, the housekeeper knew that it was her place to voice her concern and that we would respond accordingly."

Beyond Person Centered Care

The person centered approach applies to all aspects of care at Vermilion Cliffs. Indeed, the approach applied at Vermilion Cliffs moves beyond person centered care and toward a culture of person directed care, where the desires of the individual are not only at the center of the care circle but also guide caregiving. "This model demands one hundred percent employee participation and accountability," explains Ms. Mitchell. "When we have discussions about changing a system and we hear [from staff] 'It is going to interfere with my break' or 'I will not be able to finish showering five residents,' we are not happy. We want staff to understand that the choice was made for the comfort of the residents. Staff should adjust their schedules around the individual schedules of the residents. That is person directed culture."

Person directed care can result in significant improvements for individuals, with lower rates of incontinence, decreased hospitalizations, and increased satisfaction among staff members, family members, and the individuals with dementia. Director of Education and Research at Beatitudes, Tena Alonzo, describes how person directed care allows patients to bathe, sleep, and eat whenever they want, even if it is in the middle of the night.

"Generally, the person who eats what they want lives longer and in that time has a better quality of life," says Ms. Alonzo. "Most of the residents need ambulatory assistance. If a resident regularly likes to have a midnight snack, they will not be

14

up walking around and in the kitchen alone. Staff understand that addressing this habit is part of their responsibility."

Allowing residents to set their own dining schedule has additional benefits for residents, including weight gain and a reduction in medications, such as Lipitor. At Vermilion Cliffs, most residents average four medications per person, per day over the long term, including pain medications. This is lower than the national average. As Ms. Alonzo says,

> I had the opportunity to speak to the Institute of Medicine a couple of years ago. We told them about our medication rate. They were amazed. It seems like an obvious quality of life choice to us. When a person has a terminal condition and you give them many medications, they often cannot eat because they are full of medications. They also may not feel well because of the strength of the medications on their frail frame. It makes sense to start reducing the medications. We talk with families about Aricept and Namenda. The resident might have been taking medications for nine years and they might not be working much anymore, if at all. Now they are just creating expensive urine and uncomfortable stomachs.

Ms. Mitchell adds,

> We want the right drug in the right dosage for the right person for the right reason. Some people need medication, but you must investigate all medication usage. There is an experimental nature to how we view everything. We are continually examining what works and what does not. When we take a medication away, we watch closely for any positive or negative effects. We see positive effects almost always. We carefully document and observe. The documentation helps us with the inspectors, as do our favorable health outcomes. Inspectors need to be certain that we are making choices that are safer and have better outcomes for our residents.

There are ongoing positive ripple effects of reducing medications, including the need for fewer staff to administer them, fewer calls to the doctor to address issues with them, and fewer incident reports. Similar positive outcomes are seen in allowing residents at Vermilion Cliffs to sleep as long as they would like. "If you let people sleep as long as they like, they are far happier when we help them up out of bed," says Ms. Mitchell. "We need fewer staff when the resident is not angry that we woke them up and are forcing them out of bed. It is the same for eating, showering, and all other activities."

Significant benefits from person directed care have also been recorded at St. John's Home, a long-term care community in the state of New York that offers Alzheimer's and dementia care. Rebecca Priest is Administrator of Skilled Nursing at St. John's Home, where residents stay for an average of about three years. In her interview with ACCESS Health, Ms. Priest gave a comprehensive overview of how person directed care is applied by all staff on a daily basis and the impact it has on the well-being of residents. She describes one of the residents with dementia, Mr. J:

> Mr. J is a man who lives "in organization" with dementia. Living "in organization" means that residents at all stages of dementia and aging live together. The way that Mr. J's dementia has manifested is that he does a lot of searching. He looks for things. He explores places. He is continually busy. He was a marathon runner. He was an avid traveler. . .
>
> Mr. J had certain habits that were somewhat startling to people. Elders like Mr. P, who is alert and oriented, would say, "Why are you touching my hair?" Some residents would wake up from a sound sleep to find Mr. J sitting in their room. We took a deep look into how we could help Mr. J become recognized to the staff and the residents. We worked with him and

his family to determine what he needed. Mimi DeVinney is our dementia specialist. She spent time watching Mr. J, to understand his patterns and unmet needs. Mimi found that Mr. J's unmet need was touch. Touch is a very personal activity. Mimi noticed that no one was touching him proactively. She said, "Let us try something. Let us try giving Mr. J a hug when we see him. Maybe we can provide some of the human connection he is craving."

She also coached his family. His wife was taken aback because she had not touched her husband in an intimate manner in a long time. The staff hug him whenever he wants a hug. Sometimes he will walk right by and that means he does not want a hug. Instituting hugging has stopped Mr. J from touching people in search of a physical connection. It has given him a great way to make the connection he needs. Hugging also helps the staff see him differently. He has become everyone's buddy. When I hug Mr. J, we share a connection that is positive and uplifting for us both.

We wanted to create a way for people to know Mr. J when he came into the house. We made a binder with stories about him. The book shares details and photos about him in his role as an uncle. It describes him as a professional. His wife shared her story of their life together. It includes old and new stories. The book shows Mr. J as an uncle and a husband. It reminds the reader that he was an incredible professional and a marathon runner. He is no longer scary to residents when they know details about his life. He may not be able to talk about those details because they are no longer accessible to his brain. Mr. J is now seen as a man living with dementia rather than as a stranger continually strolling around.

While a passionate proponent of person directed care, Ms. Priest acknowledges the challenges in maintaining a one hundred percent person directed model due to safety and health regulations, often imposed at the state or federal level. For example, if a resident wants to smoke a cigarette on the smoke free St. John's campus, they are not permitted to. Instead, staff must create a plan for the resident to go off campus to smoke. The plan is scrutinized by the Department of Health. Similarly, if a resident wants to store food in the kitchen, staff members are obliged to ensure that the food is stored safely and only for an appropriate period of time. As Ms. Priest notes, the regulations in effect are all based on risk aversion.

Reducing Risks Associated with Dementia

Mitigating risk for people living with dementia in long-term care centers and at home is an important aspect of care that cannot be overlooked. Unfortunately, caregivers and family members often take control away from people living with dementia in a misguided effort to protect them from physical harm or other consequences.

Dr. Allen Power is a board certified internist and geriatrician, a clinical associate professor of medicine at the University of Rochester, and a Fellow of the American College of Physicians and the American Society for Internal Medicine. He is also an international educator on transformational models of care for older adults, particularly those living with changing cognitive abilities. Dr. Power explores the conflicting dynamics of safety, security, and high quality dementia care in detail in his interview with ACCESS Health.

> We tend to view the idea of safety and security through a narrow lens. It is a lens of physical safety. It is the litigious lens of preventing the worst-case scenario. I do not want to minimize anyone being hurt, but we are only seeing one side of the security

issue. I define security as supporting both emotional and psychological security. Many restraints, including locked doors, have the opposite effect. They actually make people much less secure because they cannot get out and cannot move freely. They feel trapped and often also feel that they need to get away from something that is there. As a result, we are trading one kind of safety for another kind of security and, in many cases, making people feel worse instead of better. Is the locked door really helping the residents or the providers?

Instead of locking the doors to a facility, innovative person centered care requires caregivers to first remove the stressors that make individuals want to leave in the first place. "There is no way to enable quality of life and eliminate all risk. We have to continually negotiate risk," says Dr. Power. "We have to understand that, for every person who leaves the home, there are hundreds of people who are being put on antipsychotics, who are distressed and traumatized every single day behind a locked door. They are withdrawing and giving up on life. That never makes the news. We have to balance those two."

The globally acclaimed De Hogeweyk dementia care complex applies this approach every day at their facilities, located on the outskirts of Amsterdam in the small town of Weesp. Dubbed the Dementia Village by CNN, De Hogeweyk allows all residents to roam the four acre complex freely. There are supermarkets, hair salons, theaters, and post offices, just like any other village. The shops are staffed by caretakers who wear regular clothing. There is a security system, including cameras, which monitor activities across the village. There is also only one door that leads out of the village complex and into the rest of the town. Residents who live at De Hogeweyk all live with severe dementia.

Creating Environments to Promote Autonomy and Freedom of Choice

Eloy Van Hal is one of the founding members of De Hogeweyk and one of its leading developers. "Residents live their own lives in De Hogeweyk," explains Mr. Van Hal in his interview with ACCESS Health.

> They wander or walk freely around the whole village. Everybody who is working in the village, volunteers and employees, are responsible for the residents. We all look after the residents while they are walking and wandering around. We all keep an eye on them. We support them when needed. We also invite the residents to normal daily activities such as going to the supermarket for groceries. The village model makes it possible to socialize, or to meet other people on the street or in club life. Sometimes residents even visit other houses. Sometimes they stay over for dinner. The caregivers in each house communicate with each other. After dinner, caregivers help residents find their way back home. The dementia village concept allows people to make their own choices and to meet other people with similar interests and hobbies . . . Daily life challenges individuals who suffer from severe dementia. A traditional nursing home environment or hospital is confusing and stressful. The world seems dangerous. We made people more comfortable by making their world recognizable and safer.

De Hogeweyk also made its residents healthier. Residents at De Hogeweyk live longer, eat better, and appear more joyful than those in standard long-term care facilities.

However, life at De Hogeweyk is not without risk and Mr. Van Hal acknowledges that mitigating risk is a major challenge. The De Hogeweyk complex reduces risks to residents significantly. While it operates like a true village, with open streets and neighborhood shops, it is still in the end a closed and guarded community. The long-term goal, says Mr. Van Hal, is to create an environment that is not closed off in any way and is still relatively safe for residents:

We need to work together with the community to raise awareness about dementia. Everyone should be aware of the symptoms. Once we raise awareness, we can discuss risks and risk prevention. This would enable the people with dementia to have greater personal choice and express preferences, thus improving their overall quality of life. We can build an open, dementia friendly community. We want to create an integrated village where people who do not suffer from dementia can rent an apartment. We can have a mix of individuals. In the same way we create a safe environment for children, we should create a safe environment for individuals suffering from dementia. Decades into the future, I imagine we may not even need dementia villages. Perhaps we can just create dementia friendly communities. That is a vision for the future.

Achieving that vision on a global scale may be many years away, as many local and regional governments impose restrictions on people with severe dementia walking on the streets alone. Still, at a micro level, dementia caregivers can create environments that support autonomy, personal choice, and freedom for individuals. The Hof en Heim care center in the Netherlands has created a similarly open and dementia friendly community at their Cornelia Hoeve farm. The farm houses residents in twelve beautifully renovated apartments that were once stables on the farm.

Residents are encouraged to take active part in all daily activities, such as cleaning the house, doing the dishes, and doing the laundry. They are also invited to work in the gardens around the farm, though none of these activities are forced. The caregivers at the farm follow the rhythm of the residents, providing the necessary support so residents can eat, sleep, and spend time with others as they like.

Everything on the farm is designed to make it easier for the residents to live. For example, furniture is often painted a brightly colored red. People with dementia often face significant deterioration in their sight, but bright red is one of the colors they are able to see best as their dementia progresses. Annie Herder was the manager of the Cornelia Hoeve farm for five years and now works at one of the other Hof en Heim facilities. She describes the philosophy of the farm:

> Our vision of dementia care is focused on the living environment. Scents, colors, shapes, lights, and sounds have a major effect on how people feel and behave. The brain of dementia sufferers is particularly sensitive to this. We cannot do anything about the condition, but we can control the environmental factors. That is our vision. The more pleasant the environment, the less demented the behavior. The furniture, the lights, the garden—it all looks pleasant.

Peppering the environment with familiar objects can also have an important effect on the well-being and quality of life of residents. In a 2017 interview with *The Washington Post*, the director of a nursing home in the former East German city of Dresden describes how he uses the environment to help recreate life before the fall of the Berlin Wall. His efforts began with the purchase of a 1960s-era East German motor scooter which he used to decorate the nursing home. "They remembered features of the scooter," Gunter Wolfram, the nursing home director, said of the residents. "[They] told us stories about how they had gone on trips with their friends in the past."

Wolfram went on to purchase other items that were commonly seen in communist East Germany in the 1960s, such as radios, hair dryers, and advertisements. All the items are displayed in a memory room, which is furnished according to the styles of the time and features a small supermarket stocked with items from the former German Democratic Republic. As the *Post* reports:

> Wolfram and his team of nurses soon noticed changes among patients who spent their days in an environment modeled after the Germany they had once known. They began to drink more water and eat more, and could suddenly go to the toilet again by themselves. "They showed abilities they did not show at all prior to that," Wolfram said.

Using the environment to help improve health is also a focus at elderly care facilities operated by Aleris, a private Scandinavian healthcare company with locations in Denmark, Norway, and Sweden. Linda Martin is the manager at the Aleris elder care home Odinslund in Stockholm. A focus on the living environment shapes every aspect of the Odinslund experience, even down to food, as Ms. Martin describes.

> It is important to have a calm and peaceful environment when we serve food to patients with dementia . . . Studies also show that classical music stimulates appetite. We listen to classical music when we eat to create a peaceful atmosphere that surrounds you. We also use different colors. People who suffer from dementia appreciate the contrasts on their plate. Potatoes, meat, and salad are nice colors together. The different colors of the food help our patients to understand what they are eating. One symptom of dementia is that you are unable to remember information. It is important to be concrete and distinct in the way you serve and present the food.

The Odinslund elder care home, like all the most innovative dementia care initiatives, also follows a person centered approach, in which caregivers follow the needs of the patients. The staff encourages active participation of all residents, suggesting that residents take on small responsibilities around the home, such as handing out books or making the table. Taking part in daily activities provides meaning to each resident, improves their quality of life, and helps them remain independent. If residents can remain independent, they can remain autonomous for much longer and maintain a greater freedom in life.

The Potential of New Technologies

For a person living with dementia, being able to remain in one's own home and to follow lifelong routines is possibly the greatest form of freedom and autonomy. Staying at home is often quite difficult for a person living alone as dementia progresses, due to the loss of motor skills and cognitive abilities necessary to care for oneself. When a person with dementia lives with others, the burden often becomes unmanageable for the informal caregivers, who are frequently untrained family members or close friends.

With rapid advances in technology, people living with dementia are able to overcome the hurdles presented by living at home and can often delay the move to a long-term care facility. One example of the newest technology at work for people living with dementia is IntelligentLIFE. IntelligentLIFE is an information technology system that monitors the safety and actions of an individual living with dementia and provides a communications and planning platform that connects the individual to all formal and informal caregivers that allows the caregivers and the individual to update each other on important events.

The IntelligentLIFE system uses sensor technology and complex algorithms to support people living with dementia. For example, if a person with dementia regularly wakes up in the middle of the night to use the bathroom, bed and wall sensors detect the movement and the algorithm notes the routine. Once the routine is established in the system, the next time the person wakes up to use the bathroom the system automatically turns the hallway light and bathroom light on to guide the person to the bathroom. Once the person returns to bed, the lights automatically turn off.

The system can also monitor activity in the kitchen, detecting whether a stove element has been left on too long and potentially forgotten about. In this case, the stove can be turned off remotely. By noting the routines of the individuals at the center of the care circle, the system can alert caregivers to other issues of concern. For example, if the system knows that a particular individual goes into the kitchen twice a day to prepare food and then suddenly one day they don't go into the kitchen at all, the system notifies the caregiving circle about the change and caregivers can then check on the well-being of the individual. Without this type of technology, family or friends may not be willing to leave a loved one with dementia unattended, even for important outside events. With the technology, caregivers are able to regain their own independence and leave the house knowing they will be alerted if there is any cause for concern.

The system can also detect smaller and less urgent issues at a very early stage, often earlier than a caregiver. Bo Iverson is the Sales and Marketing Manager at IntelligentLIFE. He explains,

> We can see if you are starting to become sick, if you are anxious. If your behaviors deviate thirty percent from what is normal for you, then we send an alert. We can use the design as a dialogue tool. We understand what is happening in your life. Maybe you typically go to the bathroom once a night. Now you do it four times a night. Are you getting an infection? Is something wrong? . . . One lady was in pain every day . . . She never slept more than forty minutes at a time. We alerted the care workers, who brought in the doctor. The doctor administered new medication and the lady started sleeping again.

The system also has a communication and social networking element to it. Users are given a tablet that lets them message friends and family or connect with them via video. There are calendar and task applications included that let anyone in the care circle schedule appointments and visits. The shared calendar lets everyone in the care circle know whether the individual is visiting enough with friends and family to avoid the isolation and loneliness that often comes with dementia.

Technology to Improve Overall Quality of Life

Rise Care Home is one of the long-term care facilities in Aabenraa that uses the IntelligentLIFE system. Rise Care Home employs a vast range of new technologies to improve the life of its residents. This goes well beyond the IntelligentLIFE system alone. The home has a software program called Touch and Play, which was specifically designed to support people with dementia. The residents can use the online dashboard to watch movies, play games, or use applications to help prevent cognitive decline.

Rise Care Home also invested in therapeutic robot companions for residents, in addition to real animals that residents feed and take care of. The robotic animals react to residents when they are held, calming residents when they are stressed or angry.

Gerke de Boer, who works with Annie Herder at the Cornelia Hoeve farm for people living with dementia, is incredibly optimistic about the use of robots. In the next ten years, he hopes that all residents at Cornelia Hoeve will have their own personal robots to act as companions, early detection systems, and reminders. "Robots improve life, especially for elder psychiatric individuals," says Mr. de Boer. "The robot will need to recognize if a person is sad, glad, happy, or worried. A brain that is damaged like a dementia brain can be misled easily. When they see a robot smiling, they really think it is a smiling person. That is why elderly people with a doll think it is a real baby." The robots will also help remind residents to take their medicine and exercise, and will generally keep them alert.

Coordinated Care at the Highest Level

Assisted living technologies and digital solutions are also critical to ensure the seamless coordination of care. The best practices described in the preceding pages are implemented most effectively when they are integrated under one umbrella of care, where family members, friends, doctors, nurses, and long-term care facility staff have an equal understanding of the needs and desires of the person they are caring for.

IntelligentLIFE technology has been adopted by the municipality of Aabenraa in southern Denmark. The system connects to individual municipal health records, ensuring integrated care coordination between the person with dementia, their informal caregivers, and the formal healthcare system. Aabenraa municipality has a long tradition of engaging private sector tech innovations with the care provided by the public sector health agencies. Aabenraa municipality is responsible for all local health services, including primary care, homecare, elder care, rehabilitation, psychiatric care, and the management of nursing homes and other specialized institutions. The municipality also finances twenty percent of regional healthcare services, such as hospital care. For example, if a citizen of the municipality is hospitalized, the municipality covers twenty percent of the costs of hospitalization. The incentive is then to keep citizens healthy and to inspire them to continue living active, healthy, and independent lives in Aabenraa.

Jakob Kyndal is the Director for Social Care and Healthcare in the municipality of Aabenraa. In his interview with ACCESS Health, he describes how the local government coordinates person centered care for people living with dementia, focusing private sector companies, public sector institutions, and formal and informal caregivers toward a single goal.

> We have embarked on a new mission statement that is going to focus all seventeen hundred employees in the department on the same task instead of everyone running in multiple directions. What we try to do is instill the various disciplines with the same mindset, a rehabilitating mindset focused on working together with individual citizens.
>
> We take a practically oriented approach to assisted living technology and development. We do it as part of daily business. We do not do it in labs. We let industry do that. For instance, they can go to Odense municipality to work on robots. What we try to do is simple. We do the development together with citizens. We tell industry to come to us because here we can provide a natural, practical, person centered environment where they can work directly with those who are going to use their solutions. We develop solutions together.

By sharing one common mission and working closely with the private sector to develop new innovations to coordinate care, the municipality is able to overcome the complex challenges of delivering person centered care across multiple sectors with limited funding. The approach also allows people living with dementia to live at home longer thanks to technological innovations like IntelligentLIFE.

A similar coordinated approach is applied in the Netherlands, where the Buurtzorg neighborhood model of care originated. Buurtzorg, which is Dutch for "neighborhood care," is a highly successful model of quality homecare. It was founded a decade ago by a nurse, Jos de Blok, and began with a team of just four nurses. They developed the model because they were dissatisfied with the way traditional homecare was delivered, where nurses often worked in isolation from other care providers and were burdened by heavy bureaucracy. The Buurtzorg model uses new technologies to organize care and register individuals in need. Care is then delivered by small self-managing teams made up of twelve caregivers, at most. The caregivers are often nurses. They act as health coaches for individuals in need of care and their families. The nurses focus on preventive healthcare and deliver some primary care. They coordinate more specialized care as needed. The model is now being applied by policymakers in many other countries across the world. As Mr. de Blok said in his interview with ACCESS Health,

> We need to provide healthcare staff with enough freedom to do what they think helps people. We need to work together. The current problems in healthcare are nothing that one person can solve independently. I try to involve everyone, including patients and nurses. If several people in one neighborhood struggle with the same problems, we may develop collective programs to

support these people. I think we started an important process that led to an international discussion on how we are doing this.

In short, they are simplifying the healthcare system by divorcing the financial elements of care from the delivery of care.

We disconnected the financial part from the professional part. We do not get paid for everything we do. Instead, we created an organization where the revenue is enough to cover all necessary costs. We are structured differently compared to other healthcare organizations. Our organization is flat, with fewer levels of hierarchy and lower overhead costs. At Buurtzorg, the overhead costs are eight percent, compared to twenty-five or thirty percent at the average healthcare organization. We only have well-educated healthcare workers. Our staff members design their own care methods based on what they see in the community. Our staff members each have skills in different methods. As a result, we can spend more money on the education level of nurses. We can also spend more time on networks supported by the internet and social media. We can provide healthcare to everyone, even to people without insurance or citizenship.

The cost effective approach to care offered by Buurtzorg and the other care providers described in this book is a critical necessity in dementia care. The estimated worldwide cost of dementia was 818 billion US dollars in 2016. Given that the number of people living with dementia will more than double by 2050, the costs associated with dementia care will soon be in the multi-trillions of dollars.

Support for the Informal Caregiver

Government healthcare resources can be stretched furthest if people living with dementia can extend the length of time that they remain living in their own homes. Initiatives like the Buurtzorg model and technologies like IntelligentLIFE help toward this goal, but interim homecare and new technologies are not enough to keep people with severe dementia safe and cared for at home over the long term. One of the biggest factors that influences whether a person living with dementia can remain at home is whether the person caring for them on a daily basis—the spouse, son, daughter, or friend—can continue to shoulder the heavy burden of care.

Those caring for a person with dementia are often under a great deal of pressure. They report feelings of extreme stress, frustration, depression, and loneliness as they see their loved ones become more and more distant and cognitively inaccessible. They also face the physical burden of care as the individual with dementia loses control of basic motor skills.

Supporting the informal caregiver is a cost effective and necessary intervention to ensure high quality of care for the person living with dementia. Dr. Mary Mittelman is a Research Professor in the Department of Psychiatry at the New York University School of Medicine. She developed the NYU Caregiver Intervention, which is an evidence based program that provides support to spouses, partners, and families who care for a relative with dementia. The intervention consists of four components: individual counseling sessions; family counseling sessions; weekly support group meetings; and telephone support from counselors at any time the service is needed.

"The package as a whole is crucial," says Dr. Mittelman. "For example, you cannot provide family counseling alone, even though it is the most potent ingredient . . . The NYU

Caregiver Intervention is a package and each part of the package has a contribution. It is like baking a cake. You cannot take an ingredient out and get the same cake. If you did, you would make a different cake."

The intervention has been tested and retested by Dr. Mittelman and her team over a period of more than thirty years. In one such test, NYU Caregiver counseling and support was offered to a treatment group while a control group received limited support. The results were significant.

> [T]he caregivers in the treatment group had fewer symptoms of depression. They had much less severe stress reactions to the patient's behavior despite the fact that the patient's behavior did not change. They had better self-rated health . . . We postponed nursing home placement for a year and a half longer among people whose caregivers were in the treatment group than among those in the control group. Satisfaction with social support, with emotional support from family and friends, with assistance from family and friends, and the number of people to whom the primary caregiver felt close made the difference. Those were the mediators of all the other outcomes.

The government of the United States funded the study and development of the NYU Caregiver Intervention program through its National Institute of Mental Health and, later, through the National Institute on Aging. As Dr. Mittelman notes in her interview, the government loved the outcomes from the study. Around ten years ago, the Administration on Aging asked states to apply for funding to conduct what they call "community translations" of the intervention. To date there have been more than a dozen translations and trials of the intervention conducted across the United States and in other countries, such as Australia and Israel.

The NYU Caregiver Intervention is now a proven best practice in dementia care. Indeed, all the innovations described in this opening analysis are proven practices that can improve the quality of care within the context of limited healthcare resources. Inclusive care, person centered care, person directed care, the use of technology to mitigate risks and increase autonomy and care quality, and the seamless coordination of care can and should be applied at every level when caring for people living with dementia. We encourage you to read about the specific innovations described in our analysis in the following pages, where we provide the full transcripts of our interviews with dementia care providers in the United States and Europe.

In the following pages, we include the full interviews with the experts on dementia care who are referenced above and listed here:

Advocates for Inclusion

Living with Dementia: An interview with Brian LeBlanc

Redefining Dementia: An interview with Karen Love, Jackie Pinkowitz, and Lon Pinkowitz of the Dementia Action Alliance

Person Centered and Person Directed Care

Norwegian Advisory Unit for Aging and Health: An interview with Janne Rosvik

Person Centered Dementia Care and Healthy Dying: An interview with Davina Porock

A Palliative Approach to Dementia Care: An interview with Lotta Roupe

Person Directed Dementia Living: An interview with Beatitudes Campus

St. John's Case Study: An interview with Rebecca Priest

The Living Environment

Dementia Beyond Disease: An interview with Allen Power

Dementia Village: An interview with Eloy van Hal

Dementia and Farm Life: An interview with Gerke de Boer and Annie Herder

Improving Dementia Care and Care of the Elderly: An interview with Linda Martinson

New Technologies

Elder Care Technology: An interview with Bo Iversen

Rise Care Home: An interview with Kirsten Springborg and Mette Pawlik Olesen

Aabenraa Municipality: An interview with Jakob Kyndal

Home Care

A Neighborhood Model of Care: An interview with Jos de Blok and Gertje van Roessel

Supporting the Caregiver: An interview with Mary Mittelman

Living with Dementia

An interview with **Brian LeBlanc**

About Brian LeBlanc

Brian LeBlanc is a national public speaker with Alzheimer's disease. He is an advocate for dementia awareness and education. Mr. LeBlanc is an Advisory Council member at the Dementia Action Alliance. The alliance raises awareness about what it is like to live with dementia. At the Alzheimer's Association, Mr. LeBlanc is a member of the national Early Stage Advisory Group and the local executive committee.

Mr. LeBlanc is also on the leadership board for Covenant Care. This organization develops programs and services for patients with various forms of dementia, such as Alzheimer's disease, and their loved ones. Mr. LeBlanc lives in Pensacola, Florida, with his wife Shannon and their two children.

In this interview, Mr. LeBlanc discusses his efforts to address the stigma of Alzheimer's disease and other forms of dementia. He also shares his experiences of maintaining an active and involved life with dementia.

INTERVIEW

Jean Galiana (JG): Please share your personal experience with dementia.

35

Brian LeBlanc (BL): I am the fourth generation of my family to have Alzheimer's. I am fifty-five years old. My great-grandmother had Alzheimer's. She had seven children. Of those children, one was my grandfather. One of his sisters had Alzheimer's. That sister had ten children. One was stillborn. The remaining nine all had Alzheimer's. My grandfather and grandmother had two children—my mother and my aunt. My aunt developed brain cancer. My mother had Alzheimer's. I am one of five children. I am the youngest. I am the only one that has the disease. My father had vascular dementia. My wife's grandmother passed away from Alzheimer's.

I have been around this disease since the early 1980s. I have seen the effects of Alzheimer's. When I give my presentations about Alzheimer's and other dementia related illnesses, I do not try to paint a rosy picture of it, because it is not pretty. There is nothing good about the disease, especially because there is no cure or method to slow its progression.

My friend, who is a local musician, and I sing in senior care facilities. People are horrified when I tell them that I am going to a senior care facility to sing for people with Alzheimer's. They are concerned that I will be in contact with many people with more advanced dementia. My thought is that I hope someone like me will come and sing songs to me when I am in their position. You cannot believe how it lights up their faces! Music transports people to a different time and place. Music takes you away from thinking about how you used to be and what your life used to be.

Recently, my wife and I went to see James Taylor. He is almost seventy years old. He still sounds like the James Taylor of old. The music transported me back to the 1970s and 1980s. I sat there with the biggest smile on my face because it was wonderful.

JG: In all the time you have spent around Alzheimer's, have you seen improvements in areas such as treatment, stigma, or prevention?

BL: Unfortunately, no. I will tell you why. If you talk to anyone about cancer, their response is, "Do you mean brain cancer, prostate cancer, breast cancer, pancreatic cancer, or another form of cancer?" They list all the different kinds of cancers because they know about them. They know all about cancer because there are ways to treat and possibly cure the disease. Everyone knows about HIV/AIDS, heart disease, and diabetes. When it comes to Alzheimer's, all they know is that it is the disease that old people get. We need to bring more awareness and education about Alzheimer's and other forms of dementia to the general population. Hopefully we can inspire honest conversations and slowly chip away at the pervasive stigma and fear that surrounds the disease.

JG: Is your desire to increase awareness and education what drove you to join the Advisory Council of the Dementia Action Alliance?

BL: Yes. I am also on the leadership board of Covenant Care. I am part of the national Early Stage Advisory Group of the Alzheimer's Association. Locally, I am on the executive committee of the Alzheimer's Association. I do not work anymore. My efforts are all voluntary. Dementia advocacy is what I do as a career. I want to be involved. Do you know who Sandy Halperin is?

JG: I do. But please share your thoughts about Mr. Halperin.

BL: Sandy Halperin lives in Tallahassee, Florida. Like me, he is an alumnus of the Alzheimer's Association and the Leadership Advisory Council of the Dementia Action Alliance. He also lives with Alzheimer's. He has been a committed advocate for living a vital and vibrant life with dementia.

He encouraged me to become involved in dementia advocacy and awareness. He has inspired me. I plan to take the torch from him and keep it going when the time comes. In December, I was in Washington, DC, to participate in a panel discussion at the technical conference for the American Association of Retired Persons. I told my story to a room full of guests.

JG: What else have you done as far as education and advocacy?

BL: I am a big social media geek. I have my own Facebook page strictly for Alzheimer's. It is called My Alzheimer's Journey. I have a blog entitled Alzheimer's: The Journey. I am also active on Twitter. I give many presentations around the Panhandle area of Florida. Occasionally, I travel to Mobile, Montgomery, and Birmingham, Alabama. I go everywhere that I am invited to speak.

JG: What is the message you convey in your speaking engagements?

BL: Alzheimer's is no longer a disease of the elderly. People should know the difference between dementia and dementia related illnesses. I also speak about the stigma that is associated with the disease. There is rampant stigma around Alzheimer's. People think someone with Alzheimer's cannot do anything. There are many of us with Alzheimer's who live somewhat good lives. We on the advisory board discussed stigma when we were in Washington. All twelve of us have dementia. People were surprised that we were walking around, talking, and sounding somewhat intelligent. People were asking themselves, "How can this be? This person has Alzheimer's. My grandmother has Alzheimer's and she is in a senior care facility. She cannot do anything." I explained to them that one day I will be in the same condition as their grandmother. I do not know when. Right now I am enjoying my life for the most part.

JG: You seem perfectly functional.

BL: You are seeing me on a good day. I also have plenty of bad days. Those days are difficult. My wife is helpful on the bad days.

JG: What are the characteristics of a bad day?

BL: My brain does not work well on a bad day. For the past two mornings, I have had difficulty getting started. Sometimes the difficulty lasts a little while. Sometimes it passes quickly. I can take a long time deciding what to wear. Having this appointment to talk with you helped me, because I knew that I had to shake it off and be able to talk intelligently to someone.

JG: Does getting your message out help you to focus, and therefore give you something back?

BL: Yes. Absolutely.

JG: What other benefits do you receive from all your advocacy and awareness efforts?

BL: The feedback. People come up to meet me after I speak. It makes me happy. Their comments amaze me. They regularly tell me that I am brave and speak with such passion. They are surprised I can share my story and help to dispel the stigma. I have the same response every time. I look at them and say, "How could I not do this? If I did not advocate and share my experiences, I would be sitting at home in my recliner—probably having my brain go to mush. This allows me to remain active." If I can educate and make people aware of Alzheimer's by talking to them and answering their questions, it benefits us both. It likely benefits me more than it benefits the audience.

JG: Do you think the public is taking dementia seriously enough?

BL: No. I do not mean any disrespect when I say this, but I get angry in November during football season when the National Football League is all wearing pink. I understand they are trying to raise awareness about breast cancer. But I ask myself, "Where is the purple for Alzheimer's?" With all the heads that get damaged in football leading to cognitive issues, I would think they would be wearing purple some seasons. I am going to make that my mission.

JG: Please tell me more about your blog post "The Angry Side of Alzheimer's" for the Dementia Action Alliance.

BL: That blog post was inspired by an interaction I had with my wife Shannon. One evening, Shannon and I were driving back from one of my presentations. I asked her how I did. She knows when I ask a question, I want an honest answer. She just started crying. I thought, "What did I say or what did I do?"

She said, "People get to see the polished you. They get to see who you used to be. Why do they not get to see the angry, confused, frustrated person that I see every day? Why do they not know that every morning you need migraine medication and a warm compress before you are able to speak?"

I used to work in marketing. I appeared on radio and television weekly. I cannot explain how or why, but when I get in front of an audience, the public relations guy that resides in my long-term memory comes out and takes over. I have no control over it. It just happens. It is like a light switch. When a local news station interviewed me a couple of months ago, I told them I wanted them to follow me throughout my journey with this disease. I did not want them to report only on the good days. I wanted to show people the whole picture. My wife inspired that choice.

I have always been a perfectionist. Now it is amplified. Something as simple as getting dressed can be laborious. I spend too long thinking about what to wear. There are things that I

40

used to do with ease that have become difficult. It recently took me almost a whole day to trim a bush. It used to be easy. Now I've become meticulous about every single thing. It is almost like I am super focused on the task at hand. That is not good for my family because sometimes I am too intense.

JG: Is there anything else you would like to share with our readers?

BL: I saw this quote last night on Twitter. It said something like: "My eyes can still see, my ears can hear. I am still me inside. Just know that I am still me. Do not forget me." I have lost friends, and family has become distant because of my Alzheimer's. I believe that is because they do not know how to talk to me. I guess they worry that they may say something I will not understand or ask me a question that I do not know the answer to. They do not realize that I can still function. I think that was also part of the inspiration for the "The Angry Side of Alzheimer's" blog post. My sister is the only one who communicates with me. My three other brothers do not. Maybe it is because they saw what the disease did to my mother. When my mother was in a more advanced stage of Alzheimer's, she stopped talking. She loved music. She would look at us and start to sing, but with no words—only sounds. She forgot the words, but not the tune. The tune from "The Sound of Music" meant she was happy. We had to try to make sense of a different kind of communication. I wonder if that is what my brothers think I am like now. They do not know because they do not talk to me.

JG: Have you found other social outlets through your advocacy, education, and training activities?

BL: Yes. The other members of the Alzheimer's Association Advisory Board and I talk. We all have the disease. It is comforting to talk to someone and know you can ask a question like, "When you are standing up, do you just suddenly start to fall?" Everyone will start laughing and say, "Yes, it happens to me once or twice a day." Imbalance is a symptom that we did not realize was associated with Alzheimer's. All of us have experienced it, yet we never talked about it because we did not have anyone to talk to about it. It helps us not feel so bad about everything.

JG: Did the members on the Alzheimer's Association Advisory Board become a support group?

BL: Exactly. We have similar challenges and experiences. We serve a one-year term with the advisory group. It started in July. It is going to end this June. Some of the members are already suggesting that we have a monthly conference. Hopefully, we will continue to talk to and to support each other. We can schedule our own conference calls and just meet every month or so. It does not have to be the end of everything. We can keep going. We just have to remember to call each other.

JG: I hope you will. Thank you for this discussion and for all your advocacy efforts.

BL: Thank you, too.

— END OF INTERVIEW —

Redefining Dementia

An interview with **Karen Love, Jackie Pinkowitz,** and

Lon Pinkowitz of the Dementia Action Alliance

Background

The Dementia Action Alliance is a volunteer coalition engaged in changing the understanding of and attitudes toward dementia. The coalition serves as a trusted source for conversations, education, and advocacy. The mission of the Dementia Action Alliance is to help create a world where people living with dementia can live full, productive, respected, and engaged lives, and their families and care partners are fully supported. The coalition strives to make inclusion in community life the standard for those living with dementia.

The activities of the coalition include convening and connecting people living with dementia to amplify their voices, which will better inform the policies, practices, and research that affect them. The coalition is committed to dispelling the beliefs that contribute to the stigma and discrimination of those living with dementia by promoting the "lived experience," stories of real people with dementia as they engage in life in numerous meaningful ways. The alliance also educates the public about the varieties and stages of dementia. The alliance advocates for policies, practices, and research that optimize the well-being of those living with dementia, and provides resource materials about living fully with dementia.

The Dementia Action Alliance is led by a board of directors and an advisory council of true experts—individuals living with dementia. The coalition members believe that highlighting the insights and experiences of those living with dementia is crucial to removing the barriers that prevent them from living fully inclusive, productive lives without discrimination or stigma. The Dementia Action Alliance partners with an active team of thought leaders, organizations, and communities.

The coalition has established workgroups that focus on arts and dementia, communications, optimizing well-being, and technology and dementia.

The Dementia Action Alliance is dedicated to creating person centered support for those living with dementia. The coalition developed person centered dementia values and principles that they believe will nurture the emotional, social, physical, and spiritual well-being of people living with dementia. Their video "Person Centered Matters" captures these values and principles. Other publications of the Dementia Action Alliance include "Living with Dementia: Changing the Status Quo," "Dementia Priorities Identified from a National Survey," "Dementia Care: The Quality Chasm," and "Words Matter: See ME Not My Dementia."

The Dementia Action Alliance resource center hosts links to blogs, books, Facebook pages, reports, papers and other publications, videos and films, and websites that educate a variety of audiences about dementia from a variety of perspectives.

In this interview, Karen Love, Jackie Pinkowitz, and Lon Pinkowitz describe the history of the Dementia Action Alliance. They detail their continued efforts to connect those living with dementia to community members and policymakers to help end the stigma of dementia by portraying people with cognitive challenges living purposeful and inclusive lives.

About Karen Love

Karen Love is a gerontologist and an expert in aging support and services with a specialty in dementia care. Professionally, she began as a speech therapist and transitioned into long-term care administration, serving in numerous positions, including administrator and director of dementia services. For the past sixteen years, Ms. Love has been a consultant and researcher on cultural change in long-term care settings as well as on practices that enhance the well-being of individuals living with dementia and those who care about and for them.

In 1996, she founded a nonprofit advocacy and education organization named CCAL-Advancing Person Centered Living. CCAL is a founding co-leader of the Dementia Action Alliance. The Alliance, directed by a leadership board of individuals living with dementia and mild cognitive impairment, is a national collaborative coalition dedicated to helping people live fully with dementia, supporting those who care about them, and stopping stigmatizing practices that erode well-being. Ms. Love currently serves as the executive director of the Dementia Action Alliance.

She has cofounded three national aging advocacy organizations, testified twice before the US Senate Special Subcommittee on Aging, published extensively, and spoken on national television as an advocate for the elderly.

About Jackie Pinkowitz, M.Ed.

As board chair of the Dementia Action Alliance and managing partner of Future Age, Ms. Pinkowitz focuses on enhancing person centered or person directed services, and on enhancing living in the aging and disability sectors across home, community, and residential settings. She serves as the consumer advisor to QualityHealth.com. There, Ms. Pinkowitz assists in creating national consumer centered initiatives for corporations and consults with technology application companies to advance both quality of care and quality of life. She has written numerous articles in professional, consumer, and peer reviewed publications and is a frequent speaker at national conferences and summits. Ms. Pinkowitz was a co-leader of the Retirement Research Foundation Project "Coalesce and Connect—Building a National Network of Dementia Care Voices," for which Ms. Pinkowitz and her coauthors received the 2015 Edna Stilwell Writing Award from the Journal of Gerontological Nursing. Ms. Pinkowitz served on the project management team for the National Institute of Health funded Center for Excellence in Assisted Living–University of North Carolina (CEAL–UNC) Community Based Participatory Research Project for Person Centered Care in Assisted Living in 2013. She served as vice chair of the national Center for Excellence in Assisted Living in Washington, DC, for three years and as a member of the Association of Healthcare Research Quality (AHRQ)/Center for Excellence in Assisted Living Disclosure Collaborative and the Center for Excellence in Assisted Living–University of North Carolina Community Based Participatory Research Collaborative on Medication Management. She earned her master's degree in education from Rutgers University and holds advanced certification in special needs populations.

About Lon Pinkowitz

Lon Pinkowitz serves on the Dementia Action Alliance board of directors. He focuses on advancing healthcare management and long-term care services through emerging technologies and person centered approaches. As a consultant, Mr. Pinkowitz applies his expertise in sales and marketing, marketing communications, and organizational systems to assist startup companies. He worked for Tsumura International as vice president of New Business Development/International Sales and Marketing. Lon has a master's degree in personnel and counseling from New York University.

INTERVIEW

Jean Galiana (JG): What inspired you to create the Dementia Action Alliance?

Karen Love (KL): I worked in a nursing home as a nursing aide when I was in high school. That experience underpinned what has become my life passion. I fell in love with the residents. I was especially drawn to older people with dementia. I would ask myself why we were not helping them up to dress in the morning. I also wondered why we were not involving them in activities or making efforts to connect with them. I was a bright eyed eighteen-year-old and was deeply concerned about older people being left out. The nursing home management wanted bathing to be done in the morning. I began sneaking people in for an evening shower because they did not want to bathe in the morning. I felt the residents with dementia were treated in a dehumanizing manner.

When I was in graduate school at George Washington University, I worked for the healthcare services graduate program's long-term care program. We searched for models of best practice in dementia care. In the late eighties and early nineties, there were not many available. The British geriatric psychologist Tom Kitwood was leading the cause and is now considered the father of person centered dementia care internationally. He innately knew how to connect with people living with cognitive impairments. He published important findings that influenced dementia care thereafter.

I then began to manage assisted living facilities. At that time, trying to run a person centered assisted living residence was like living in the Wild West. I felt the need to organize some like-minded industry professionals to explore how the industry could make important changes as a group. I launched a national consumer advocacy organization named the Consumer Consortium for Assisted Living.

Jackie Pinkowitz's mother was living with dementia in an assisted living home in Michigan. Three years later, Jackie's father-in-law was diagnosed with Alzheimer's. My father also had been diagnosed with Alzheimer's. Our personal experiences made us dedicated to change dementia care and fight the stigma of dementia.

Jackie Pinkowitz (JP): The Dementia Action Alliance is mission driven. That is why we use the tagline, powered by people with purpose. I like to say, powered by people with purpose and passion.

KL: We created the consortium at the beginning of the increase in the elderly population in the United States. Nursing homes were not prepared to care for the increasing number of people with dementia. Nursing homes were not properly regulated. I remember stories of abuse and neglect in long-term care facilities.

Eventually we witnessed significant advances like the Omnibus Reconciliation Act (OBRA) in 1987. Shortly after the act passed, regulations were established that limited the number of residents in each room to three or fewer. I know that does not sound impressive, but before the act passed, some nursing homes had six people living in one room. Only minor attention was given to special diets. There was little dementia specific training. Pharmacists would review medications only every three months.

We collaborated with then senator John Breaux. He saw the wisdom in our mission. With our urging, he and his staff succeeded in bringing the top industry players together. The consortium was composed of providers, advocates, and physicians. They began an eighteen-month period of growth and development. We were one of the few groups that were actively advocating for person centered long-term care. It was a big challenge because there were many old fashioned thinkers in the industry. Eventually we became disruptive in productive ways. Over the years, we shifted our focus and our activities to person centered dementia living.

JG: What led you to survey the national dementia funding priorities among caregivers and those living with dementia?

KL: The National Alzheimer's Project Act (NAPA) was passed in 2011. It was the first time the United States brought people together to address Alzheimer's disease, but not dementia. The act was focused mostly on a cure for Alzheimer's. We thought they should include all dementias and fund support for those living with dementia and their caregivers. That is when we drafted our white paper entitled Dementia Priorities Identified from a National Survey. The survey found that people with dementia and their caregivers wish that more national spending was devoted to supporting them in their daily lives.

JP: The National Alzheimer's Project Act was the catalyst to our forming the Dementia Action Alliance. There was no national discussion about the millions of individuals who were trying to help family members with dementia. We founded the Dementia Action Alliance to help the families and those living with dementia receive support and services. Our focus is care more than cure.

KL: We were disheartened that the government built a federal advisory council of researchers and clinicians that did not include anyone living with dementia.

JG: How do you include those living with dementia in the Dementia Action Alliance?

JP: Karen and I were committed to the concept, "nothing about us without us," from the very beginning of the Dementia Action Alliance. The expression comes from the disability world. I used to teach special needs children, and later my mother developed Alzheimer's, so I had that philosophy and mindset. We knew that the voices of those living with dementia were not being heard anywhere that mattered. We created an advisory council entirely of people living with dementia.

Karen and I realized the importance and value of having those living with dementia involved in all public and private organizations in the field of dementia. We built a national collaborative that enables people living with dementia to connect virtually and talk to one another around the world to share their insights and issues.

JG: Tell me about your workgroups.

KL: The people whom we coalesce participate in a variety of workgroups that reflect their specific areas of leadership. There is at least one person living with dementia in every workgroup. Their perspective is crucial. They offer insights and solve issues from their unique vantage point. What could be better? I do not know why every organization dealing with any aspect of dementia does not include those living with dementia. They are an invaluable resource.

We also connect those living with dementia to policymakers on the federal, state, and community levels. Last year, Sandy Halperin, the well-known advocate who is living with dementia, met with Kathy Greenlee, who is the assistant secretary of the Administration for Aging.

People living with dementia also need to be included in society. As their condition progresses, a person living with dementia loses the ability to self-initiate. That is often the reason why those living with dementia are not doing anything. They are inactive not because they do not want to be active, but because they need to be kick started through engagement. Inclusion and involvement is better for their health. It is better for their overall well-being. Many basic needs of people living with dementia, such as engagement, go unmet.

JG: Other countries began the aging expansion before the United States. Are they ahead of us in regard to dementia support and care?

KL: David Cameron convened the first G8 Summit on Dementia. The government of the United Kingdom appropriated a fair amount of funds toward dementia care. The government did not direct the funding. They gave the awards to good people on the ground level to direct it.

JG: Were the outcomes tracked?

KL: Yes. The Joseph Rowntree Foundation conducted the evaluation. Dementia Friendly United Kingdom is a robust initiative. Dementia Friendly began there because they lead the world in the growth of the older population. Japan is also producing innovative robotic products for the elderly.

JG: Are you referring to PARO the seal?

KL: If you have ever seen someone with PARO the seal, they love it. Japan is also developing other sophisticated robotics besides PARO.

JG: Please describe your thoughts about transitioning to a bio-psycho-social-spiritual culture.

KL: Atul Gawande speaks beautifully about the bio-psycho-social-spiritual culture. He believes that we have been wrong about how we imagine healthcare. We think healthcare is about safety and physical health. Our focus should be well-being. Well-being cannot be realized through physical health alone. Well-being includes biology, psychology, and spirituality—the bio-psycho-social-spiritual paradigm. Spirituality does not have to be religion. It can be watching a beautiful sunset. Spirituality is whatever touches your heart. All of these dimensions make up our well-being, especially for someone with dementia. I have done a lot of research over the years on engagement. Much of the brain remains unused. When we connect with someone or do something that is fun, part of the brain has the power to release neurotransmitter chemicals that make us happy. There are ways of connecting through those windows to reach people with dementia.

JP: These methods of connection need to be researched in depth and practiced by everyone involved, from the patient's family to the hospital that treats them. Education and awareness can inspire inclusion for those living with dementia in all settings, including the clinic and the neighborhood.

KL: The United States, and much of the world, is focused largely on the biological component of well-being. We use an acute healthcare model to treat a long-term condition. We are trying to respectfully disrupt the beliefs, attitudes, and practices about dementia in our country.

JP: We work to make the invisible visible.

JG: What do you view as invisible, regarding dementia?

JP: The spending practices that prioritize finding a cure, but neglect the needs of the caregiver and those living with dementia; the stigma that exists around dementia; and the need for dementia friendly communities and businesses.

JG: What activities are you involved with that address those issues?

KL: Caring Conversations is one.

JG: Please describe Caring Conversations.

JP: We host friendly, informal gatherings of approximately thirty people. They include people living with dementia, family caregivers, residents of the community such as police officers and shop owners, and clinicians. We meet for an hour and a half. It is a facilitated conversation. Caring Conversations is a friendly platform for the participants to share their thoughts about issues regarding dementia. Caregivers may share their challenges and methods that can help others. Providers and others hear and see people with dementia differently after these conversations. Many people have the misperception that all dementia is end stage. Those living with dementia interact with the members in the group, which helps the others to see the person before the disease. People from the gathering may leave the conversation thinking, "There is the artist," rather than, "There is the woman suffering from dementia."

Lon Pinkowitz (LP): We have also hosted pharmaceutical company executives who are developing a product for dementia. They interacted with and learned directly from their end user. Before the conversation, they were far from understanding how a person can live well with dementia. That was an important conversation.

JG: Something as simple as facilitating a conversation could potentially affect the development of particular drugs or influence the motivation behind the development?

JP: Yes. We hope that it also stimulates community champions who will be inspired to host Caring Conversations on a regular basis. The conversations can be about a variety of subjects, for example how to make the community more dementia friendly. This needs to happen not only through the built environment, but through creating person to person, human connections. Anyone is welcome to contact us if they would like to host a Caring Conversation in their community. We will support and guide their efforts.

KL: Here is one of our conversations in Washington, DC. The daughter of a woman living with dementia is speaking.

Dementia presents differently for each individual. I think the scary thing, for people who have loved ones and friends with dementia, is the unknown. You do not know how it is going to affect each person. I think the unknown is very scary. If you have a friend who is going through breast cancer, you know what to expect because there is a mastectomy, there is radiation, there is chemotherapy. Maybe their hair will fall out. Dementia, it is different case by case. I spoke with people whose grandparents had dementia and whose parents had dementia. One woman told us, "We loved it when my grandfather got dementia because he was a really mean guy before, but with dementia he was the sweetest person ever." We spoke with someone else who had a completely different experience. Another issue is that people do not know what to say to a person who has dementia.

We select our conversation group carefully. We hosted a Caring Conversation in Washington because there are many people working on the federal level, who make policies and national decisions, who do not understand what it is like to live with dementia. We invited them to have a conversation with five people living with dementia. The person who sat next to the daughter who just spoke is a pharmaceutical executive. Another participant is a senior executive vice president from AARP National. We had two chief executive officers and long-term care service providers. Forty-two people participated in that Caring Conversation. Their chairs were arranged in a large horseshoe shape so everyone could see one another.

LP: No one wanted to leave.

KL: Yes, we got kicked out of the space we had rented.

LP: We could have been in there for two days. No one wanted to stop talking.

KL: It was a two-hour conversation. It showed us that there is a need and a desire for this type of interaction. We hope to have Caring Conversations all over the country. The conversation is important, but what the participants choose to do with the new knowledge is more important. The conversations plant the seeds within the community. We facilitate connections and collaborations. We establish a small community think tank, of sorts, that focuses on dementia. The conversation participants take the lead thereafter.

JP: They take the message to the street. They know that they can always reach out to us. It is surprising how many calls Karen and I receive from people everywhere. We are always available to listen with an open heart. Sometimes the conversation participants need our expertise and support. Sometimes they just wish to maintain a relationship with like-minded people.

KL: We can validate their concerns about dementia or their struggles with dementia because we have been there ourselves and our advisory council is made up of people living with dementia.

JP: Another component of the Caring Conversation is that we want to encourage people to create a Caring Wishes notebook. Often it is difficult for someone with dementia to communicate wishes regarding their care plan and their lifestyle choices. We would like to help them document their wishes regarding their quality of life when considering future care and living options. Sandy Halperin helped us create the template. As I mentioned earlier, he is living with dementia and has been a longtime advocate for those with dementia.

JG: How does the Caring Wishes notebook process work?

KL: We offer a guide to starting the care plan discussion and provide the template during the Caring Conversations.

JG: Please tell me about the North American Dementia Education Conference.

KL: We are aligned with organizations doing important work in dementia and with those living with dementia. Because of that, we decided to create opportunities for idea sharing and collaboration. We will host the first conference in 2017 in Atlanta, Georgia.

JG: Have you chosen the areas of focus for the conference?

JP: There will be a technology track because we have a technology workgroup.

KL: Other areas of focus will include arts and dementia, optimizing well-being, and meaningful engagement. We called the conference North American because we have connections in Canada who we wish to include. The Canadian province of Ontario has many person centered dementia care initiatives. Some of the other provinces do not. The Canadian government funds are directed toward those living with dementia and not solely toward finding a cure. Our government directs only a smattering of funding through the US Administration on Aging and the Health Resources and Services Administration toward supporting those living with dementia and their formal and informal caregivers. The large majority of funding is allocated to research to find a cure.

JP: If we ask what matters most to the people living with dementia and their families and friends, the answers are simple and basic. They want relationships and connections with their families, friends, and clinical care teams.

LP: We want healthcare clinicians to understand that people living with dementia are people first and patients second. If we keep referring to them as patients, we are going to think about them as patients. Clinicians need to consider the whole person and their life, rather than only focusing on what is physically wrong and how to fix it.

KL: We are a smaller organization and need to dedicate our efforts where we can make an impact. We spent two years with the National Quality Forum on various work committees advocating for dementia care. We made a little bit of progress. For example, they were using the term "Alzheimer's" exclusively, and they agreed to change it to "dementia including Alzheimer's."

LP: It took a long time before they would make that change.

KL: We realized we were not helping a lot of people by putting our efforts in that direction. Now we are working on the community level. We think the change will come from grassroots community organizations instead of us banging on doors in Washington.

JP: We have not walked away from advocacy completely. We are still actively involved in multiple forums around dementia.

KL: We have three seats on the Dementia Friendly America initiative.

JG: Please describe the Dementia Kindness Challenge.

JP: It is a social media challenge.

KL: Brian LeBlanc, who is one of our board members living with dementia, runs the social media for the Dementia Action Alliance. People living with dementia, their friends, or their families can make a video and upload it. The video will be short and will be about their family or themselves. They will share personal experiences and then say something like, "I want you to know that Alzheimer's does not define me. I am still myself with additional challenges. I am taking the Dementia Kindness Challenge by uploading this video to YouTube, donating ten dollars for the challenge to promote awareness, and challenging someone I know to take the challenge to spread kindness." The Dementia Kindness Challenge is affirmation for people living with dementia that dementia does not define them. They are still themselves. That is powerful. It is educational. It is awareness.

JP: The Dementia Kindness Challenge contests the stigma of dementia by pulling the issue out of the shadows and shining a light on the faces of the people directly and indirectly affected by the disease. It reminds us that few are immune. We will all either have dementia or have family or friends living with dementia. We are all in this together, so let us remove the stigma.

JG: What are the challenges for the Dementia Action Alliance?

JP: If we had more partners for funding, we would hope to launch a national public awareness campaign.

JG: Is the lack of funding what is preventing you from launching the campaign?

KL: Without a doubt.

LP: That is ninety-five percent of what is holding us back.

JP: We want to change the national attitude about dementia.

KL: We want to put a face on dementia and engage those living with dementia to be the spokespeople. We would love to give more national attention to the Brian LeBlancs and Sandy Halperins who are living throughout the country.

JP: Let them speak for themselves.

KL: Yes. After all, they are the experts.

JP: We want to increase our funding to establish a larger presence. We would like to have a presence in every major convention, including some state conventions. With host partners, we could potentially facilitate Caring Conversations in communities across the US. We want to be a support, an educator, and a facilitator. We also want to inspire advocacy on the community, state, and federal levels.

KL: People want to be involved. They just need to know how. That is where we come into the picture.

JG: Who funds the Dementia Action Alliance?

JP: We are funded mostly by grants from foundations. We established the virtual infrastructure, the foundational papers, and resources that make us credible and impactful, and as a result, fundable. The Retirement Research Foundation spurred us on by telling us, "There is no one trying to connect and bring together people living with dementia so that their voices and their choices can be heard." That was when we changed the name and the focus of the organization, about five years ago. We realized we could make the most impact through our focus on dementia because of this fast growing demographic.

KL: No organizations were hosting national leadership discussions. In 2012, the Consumer Consortium for Assisted Living convened the first Thought Leader Summit on dementia. Our organization, the Eden Alternative, the Pioneer Network, Planetree, and the American Medical Directors Association made up the steering group. We had sixty people at our first Thought Leaders Summit. We began to develop the operational framework for person centered dementia care. At the time, the concept was groundbreaking.

Now, the Dementia Action Alliance is a collaboration of volunteers who embrace our vision and mission. Anyone who has an interest in making our nation a better place to live with dementia and in supporting those who are caring for someone living with dementia is welcome to be a Dementia Action Alliance partner.

JG: Tell me about the Compassionate Touch initiative.

KL: The Administration on Aging (AOA) sponsored one of the projects that I led called Compassionate Touch and Reiki. We taught Compassionate Touch to two hundred and fifty aides of a nonprofit homecare agency. Some aides were transgender because there is a population of transgender people in the district who want to have aides like themselves. Classes were given to twenty aides at a time. We had thirteen classes. Compassionate Touch is simple. It is not the hand massage that you receive when you are having your nails done. Compassionate Touch is about being with the person and the gentleness of holding someone's hand. It can accompany companionable silence or a little bit of discussion. We teach the touch points for the hands and the arms to create a relaxed, happy feeling. After the training, seventy-five aides volunteered to take their learning a step further by registering for level one Reiki practitioner training. The level one training is an hour. This nonprofit organization brought their aides in three times a year for additional training. This is unusual because the organization must pay the aides when they are not working. We taught more than the massage techniques. We taught engagement and connection.

I will never forget one aide in particular. Her name is Patricia Simms. She was the one in the class who appeared to be disinterested. To engage her, I gave her a leadership role. By the end of that training session, she shared her experience of Compassionate Touch and engagement with a woman for whom she was caring. Patricia said, "Let me tell you about this one client I have. She had been in the hospital for over a week and could not walk when she got home, so she was in a wheelchair. I knew she would be frail and weak. The training taught me to think about what I could use to build her strengths and work toward her abilities, not her limitations. I had taken her outside in her wheelchair, and we were pushing down the sidewalk. No one was paying any attention to us, and all of a sudden I said, 'OK, Mrs. B, my turn.' Mrs. B looked up at me and asked what I meant. I told her that it was my turn for a ride. I had given her a ride, now she should give me a ride. Because Mrs. B knew she had the wheelchair to hold on to while walking, she agreed and I helped her navigate around the chair. Then I sat in the wheelchair. Mrs. B had lived in the neighborhood for a long time. All the people who had previously passed and paid no attention heard the two of us laughing. People asked for a ride for themselves and told us it looked fun. They were engaging with Mrs. B. It was an entirely different interaction. This was not only fun, it got Mrs. B to exercise and become stronger faster." Patricia added, "I visited Mrs. B daily because she had just been released from the hospital. Every morning when I arrived, after our wheelchair switcheroo, Mrs. B was sitting by the front door. She could not wait to go out. She was motivated. She had gotten herself out of bed."

JP: She had something to look forward to.

KL: Yes. It was unscientific and anecdotal, but Patricia told us, "I have taken care of many people who have come out of the hospital, and it takes a long time to get them up and walking again. Mrs. B was up and walking within ten days."

Another aide who participated in the training described how she used Compassionate Touch with an ornery older woman who had arthritis in her knees. This woman hated to get out of bed. The aide remembered that warmth was the heart of the Compassionate Touch training. She would tell the older woman, "Oh Mrs. L, let us get those knees massaged. It will take some of the pain away." The aide did some gentle massage. Then the client would swing her legs around and get up. The aide told us, "I would spend an hour trying to get her out of bed before. This was motivating in a whole new way." There is some placebo effect, but warmth, touch, and connection trigger different parts of the brain, so it is not necessarily just placebo.

Mrs. L felt like she was cared for. This simple process is free and does not take long. No specialists were involved, and Mrs. L was ready to get out of bed. We know these trainings have an impact. We are seeking funding and partners to train as many health providers and volunteers as possible. The plan and strategy of the Dementia Action Alliance is to grow a bigger base so we can bring our various initiatives to more people. We also want to share the stories that remind us that it is about human connection and that dementia has a human face. What we teach is person centeredness. That is what all care is about. Stop just doing, and be present in a real way. We have heard many success stories from those trainings.

JG: Did you only do the Compassionate Touch training once as an experiment or do you conduct trainings regularly?

KL: The United States Administration on Aging funded only that one pilot program. We think that they should fund the next translation. We made an impact. Our challenge is how to bring this training to many more people.

JG: Thank you for this interesting discussion and your dedication to dementia.

JP: Thank you for your interest in our work.

LP: Thank you.

KL: Thank you for spreading the mission of the Dementia Action Alliance.

— END OF INTERVIEW —

Norwegian Advisory Unit for Aging and Health

An interview with **Janne Rosvik**

About Janne Rosvik

The research of Janne Rosvik focuses on person centered care. Rosvik has built on the previous thinking of both Tom Kitwood and Dawn Brooker. Tom Kitwood wrote about personhood and the importance of assuming the perspective of the individual who receives care; Dawn Brooker created the VIPS (values, individuality, perspective, and social inclusion) framework, which articulates Kitwood's care philosophy. Janne Rosvik has developed the VIPS practice model.

INTERVIEW

My name is Janne Rosvik. I live in Oslo, Norway. I am a registered nurse. I also have a master's degree in political science and a PhD in person centered care and dementia care. Both of my degrees are from the University of Oslo. I developed the VIPS practice model as part of my PhD research. VIPS stands for values, individuality, perspective, and social inclusion.

The V stands for the values of person centered care. The main value is that the person with dementia and the perspective of that person are just as important as our own

63

perspectives as caregivers. The I is for individual care, which means we observe and note each person's unique traits. What is special about this person? What are his habits? What other illnesses does he have? The P is for the perspective of the person with dementia. How does the world look from his point of view? The S is for social inclusion. Are his social needs taken care of? Is he included in social fellowship with other people? Each letter has six subindicators, which are used in the analysis that is part of the VIPS practice model. We check all twenty-four indicators and determine if any one of those is relevant to a given situation.

We look for several indicators. Is the external environment here good for the person? Is there something in the environment that is disturbing him? Do we care about his perspective? Are his human rights taken care of? The I, P, and S indicators are used most because they are more concrete, but we do not skip any of the four elements. This is how we make sure that person centered care is the focus here.

I have worked here in Oslo at the National Advisory Unit for Aging and Health for six years. Before that I was a lecturer in the bachelor's degree program for registered nurses. I used to work as a registered nurse and as a manager in homecare services.

When I was teaching students and preparing them for their first training period with old people in care homes, I became interested in research. About eighty percent of people living in care homes here have dementia, so most of the students' residents by far would require special care. I insisted that the program not just focus on basic nursing, but also on dementia training. The focus before was on basic nursing, personal hygiene, and nutrition. The students weren't prepared. They had to learn something about dementia care.

In my time as a practicing nurse, I found that I had a special heart for people with dementia. I like being with them. I visited those people when I was a nurse. If there were people with dementia, I volunteered to be responsible for them. It provoked a lot of thought when I talked with them. Having dementia goes to the heart of who you are as a human being. They have to battle with big existential questions. Who am I when my brain is not working well?

Another institution asked the nursing college to send some teachers to teach elder care in China. My employer sent me and another lecturer. In China, as in most of the third world, there is no tradition of care homes because they care for their elderly at home. In the big cities they have the same problem as we do in the western world: there are no people at home to give care. Both the husband and the wife are working, so there is no one at home to care for their elderly. They now recognize a need for care homes in China, but they need to teach their healthcare professionals how to care for people who are old.

When I went back to teach again, I noticed that there were no people with dementia in the care homes. When I asked them about this, they said, "We cannot admit people with dementia. They are too hard for us to handle. They do things that we cannot deal with. We do not have the skills to care for persons who are dying or for persons who are too ill."

I said, "But those two groups are the most important groups. If you cannot take in the terminally ill and people with dementia because you lack skills, then I will provide those skills." I changed the program to include those two areas. Then I developed a new program to teach those two areas specifically. As I returned year after year and visited the same places, I saw that they had started to admit people with dementia. They now know better how to care for them.

I taught all over China. I went there for nine years in a row and visited places all over the country. Back in Oslo, I started focusing more and more on dementia to prepare for my teaching in China. I started looking for literature. I found

Tom Kitwood's writings. I was fascinated by person centered care and made that the main topic of my doctoral research.

Sofia Widén (SW): What is at the core of person centered care?

Janne Rosvik (JR): The core of person centered care is to think of a person with dementia as a person who has the same needs as everybody else. The thing that is happening in his brain does not change his value as a person. It makes him a person with problems in the brain. His feelings and his emotions are still there, maybe even a bit stronger. When the person becomes agitated, which we often see, it may be because he is unable to express himself. We need to learn how to use all the knowledge we have about the symptoms of dementia to try to understand the person's perspective on the world around him. What is happening in his brain often makes it difficult for him to explain with words, so he may have to use other means of communication. It is our responsibility to learn his way of communicating. We don't just try to make this person nonaggressive; we try to understand him.

Tom Kitwood has given us a way of thinking that can help our understanding. We focus on the need for inclusion, the need for comfort, and other basic psychological needs. We look for physical needs and for pain. We cannot change the person with dementia—we have to change the focus of our care. This person is saying something sensible, like he always has. He is just struggling to say it. We have to learn how to understand each person, do the research, talk to the person, and figure out what he is trying to communicate.

Kitwood developed dementia care mapping as a way of observing how a person with dementia is doing during the day. An example of feedback from dementia care mapping might be, "This person was sitting alone for three hours, sometimes crying. When someone sat down with her, she responded very well to communication." That kind of thing. Dementia care mapping has continued to develop, but we need more methods we can use to teach healthcare personnel person centered care.

SW: Please describe dementia care mapping in more detail.

JR: You must take some courses to become a certified mapper. It is a structured way of observing a person's mood and engagement. There are fifteen categories, which you rate within a range of minus five to plus five. You watch two or three individuals for three to six hours and you record what is happening. You do not go into private rooms. You sit in a common area like the living room or the lounge. If the person is just sitting there, there is a code for that. Is he engaging in something or not? How is his mood? You use the categories to record what happens. You might see that a caregiver comes and sits down and talks to the person, and you can record that his mood goes up and his engagement rises. You record how long this activity goes on. You record what happens to the person's mood and engagement when the caregiver leaves, and so on.

After the observation (the mapping), you give feedback to the staff about your observations. Then you discuss with them what can be done. If the person responds well to something, they may decide to do more of that activity. You use mapping to discover how to help a person have a good day by noting how he fares in a variety of situations. There should be a natural flow of moods throughout the day. You can do a new mapping later to see if the intervention the staff implemented after the previous mapping session worked as intended.

SW: Do many care homes use this in Norway?

JR: Norway is one of the countries where mapping is most used.

SW: Are there disadvantages to dementia care mapping?

JR: You need to keep the knowledge present in your head. All fifteen categories. It is a lot of information. It is also very intense to sit for three to six hours and mark what is going on every five minutes. It takes time to prepare to do it, to analyze it, and then to present it. I would not say it takes too much time, but it is demanding. You need to do it frequently to be good at it.

SW: Where can you receive training in dementia care mapping?

JR: Designated persons are certified to train. It is an international network. There is a headquarters in the United Kingdom at Bradford University.

SW: Was the VIPS practice model developed here in Norway?

JR: Yes, I developed VIPS in my PhD thesis. I think dementia care mapping is a very good tool, but I wanted something additional. It was very important that it be easy to learn. The VIPS practice model is easy to learn, but once you learn it the real training begins. With the VIPS practice model, you can send a few caregivers from each unit for a course, but then the rest of the staff in the unit needs an introduction, and all of the staff needs to work together from then on. It is not like dementia care mapping, where one or two receive the training and do it independently. The whole staff uses the VIPS practice model.

We hold a weekly meeting in which everyone has a role. There is one staff member who represents the majority of the staff. This person is the chair of the meeting. If registered nurses are the majority, the chair will be a registered nurse. If assistant nurses are the majority, one of them will chair the meeting. The leader of each unit has to be present, as well as the primary contact for the resident whose care is discussed at the meeting. We also have a VIPS practice model coach in each institution who helps the staff get a good start while the VIPS practice model is new to them. Those are the main roles. The primary contact for each person is supposed to speak on behalf of the person who receives care and present the situation from his perspective.

The hub of the VIPS practice model is this weekly consensus meeting. At the meeting, each primary contact addresses the chair and says, for instance, "I would like to discuss the morning care situation for my patient." They need to discuss just one situation—not the whole person, just the morning care procedure, for example.

There is obviously something this person is trying to communicate that the caregiver does not understand. We need to discuss that. In the meeting, the caregiver is asked by the chair to tell the others what she thinks happens in this situation. How does the individual experience it, based on his facial expression and what he is saying? We encourage caregivers to interpret signals. Does he look angry? Does he look scared? Does he look frustrated? Is there some word that he is repeating? Is there something disturbing him? What does his body language say? Does he try to grab you or does he push you away? What is his perspective on the situation? This is very difficult, so we spend a lot of time training and focusing on that. We use films to teach staff how to look for signs. We have some very good films produced in England that help us take that perspective.

When the primary contact has presented the situation from the perspective of the individual, the other nurses describe how they perceive the situation. You receive as much information as you can. Then you use the VIPS framework with all the indicators and determine which indicators are relevant.

SW: How often do you recommend meetings about one

person? Is it only when issues arise, or are they scheduled regularly?

JR: If we focus on two indicators and make some interventions to improve the situation, then we typically evaluate these after a week. Did it improve the situation? If it did not, then we have to reassess.

SW: Is it challenging to make time for these meetings?

JR: Homes have to find time, and they do. They do not all find time every week, but maybe every other. The staff love the meetings because they want to do a better job. The V, for values, goes for the staff as well. They are valued too.

It is very difficult if one person says, "We need to change our routine," but the rest of the staff says, "Why should we?" But if you sit in a meeting and you conclude together that you need to change the routine to meet a person's needs, then everybody is on board. It is very difficult to change routines without the consensus of the whole group.

In Kitwood's 1997 book, *Dementia Reconsidered*, there is a chapter called "The Caring Organization." Three of the main elements from this chapter are teamwork, supportive leadership, and coaching or guidance. You can recognize these elements in our model. Teamwork is in the meeting. Supportive leadership is in the presence of a leader. That is important because she is there to support, not to lead and coach. The VIPS framework is Dawn Brooker's. She is the coauthor of two or three of my papers.

SW: Please describe the effect of person centered dementia care on quality of life measurements.

JR: In The Effects of Person Centered Dementia Care, we tested the effect of dementia care mapping and the VIPS method using the Brief Agitation Rating Scale, the Neuropsychiatric Inventory (NPI), the Cornell Scale for Depression and Dementia, and the Quality of Life in Late Stage Dementia Scale (QUALID).

We did not find a significant effect on the Brief Agitation Rating Scale with either method. We saw significant effects on neuropsychiatric symptoms with both methods. When we looked at the twelve items on the NPI (depression, agitation, irritation, sleeping disturbances, psychosis, hallucinations, delusions, and so on) we found significant reductions in all of those compared to the control group. When we looked at the subscales—one agitation subscale, one subscale for psychiatric symptoms such as hallucinations and delusions, plus another one for mood—we also found significant reductions compared to the control group.

There was a reduction in depression for both methods, but the reduction was only significant for the VIPS practice model, not for dementia care mapping. Usually depression and quality of life are parallel. If one goes up the other goes up; if one goes down the other goes down. It was very unexpected that both methods did not have a significant effect on both.

Dementia care mapping had a significant effect on quality of life and the VIPS practice model had a significant effect on depression. I think it has to do with the point of contact. In dementia care mapping, the observations were done in the eating lounge, so it focused on what was happening at the meal. The feedback was centered on things that had to do with the meal, which corresponded with some of the items on the QUALID scale.

In the VIPS practice model, the points of contact were in the individuals' rooms, not in the common areas. The focus was often on situations that corresponded with some of the items on the depression scale.

SW: What are your recommendations for the future based on these results?

JR: We think this indicates that person centered care can decrease agitation. We always thought this was the case, but it is difficult to prove. The fact that we were able to observe significant results is exceptional because this is a psychosocial intervention and very difficult to measure with a randomized control study. That is the reason why it is so difficult to say that person centered care works. So many factors can be compounded. Dementia care mapping is the method that has been researched most because it was developed two decades ago. The VIPS practice model is new.

SW: In terms of these models and your results, what would you recommend to caregivers today?

JR: We have just published a booklet called Implementing Person Centered Care. We recommend using four methods at the same time. Two of these methods are dementia care mapping and the VIPS practice model.

SW: Can you describe the other two methods?

JR: They do not spring from Kitwood's work, but the theory they use is very compatible with Kitwood's. Marte Meo focuses on micro-communication, the communication between the individual and the nurse. They use video cameras. They take three to five minutes of film of a difficult situation, then they analyze it. They determine what is happening and how the nurse can change her way of communicating. When you see it on film, things that you are not able to see when you are in the middle of it become very clear. They coach staff based on these films. It is very revealing.

SW: What is the fourth method?

JR: It is a planning tool. When we decide something in the consensus meeting in the VIPS practice model, then we have plans for the day shift regarding who does what when and the same for the night shift. How does the week look? What kind of group activities have we got during the week? These kinds of things. The plans are a way of making sure that everything is fit into the routine. That way people know what to do and when to do it.

All the methods work very well together. They do not overlap, but they reinforce each other. We tested this in two care homes. They used all the methods for nine months. They found it possible to use them all, even with our limited resources. It is not too expensive, but you have to prioritize it.

SW: Do you now train nurses in these four methods?

JR: We have courses to train them in three of these methods. We train people in conducting courses in the VIPS practice model so they can go to other institutions and train the staff there. We train the trainer.

SW: What are the key research questions that still need to be answered?

JR: They are many. How can you be a person centered leader? What should the leader do to implement person centered care and maintain focus on it? The use of these methods in homecare is also very important. These are methods that can be used outside an institution as well.

SW: Thank you for your time.

— END OF INTERVIEW —

Person Centered Dementia Care and Healthy Dying

An interview with **Davina Porock**

About Davina Porock

Davina Porock is vice provost for Faculty and Administration at Lehman College, City University of New York, in the Bronx. She has practiced nursing and has performed research in Australia, where she received her training and formal education, as well as in the United Kingdom and the United States. Dr. Porock holds adjunct professorships at the Universities of Nottingham and Canterbury Christchurch in the United Kingdom, the University of Malaya, in Malaysia, and at the University of Missouri and SUNY Buffalo in the United States.

Most of Dr. Porock's work has been in the care of older adults approaching the end of life. She is particularly interested in understanding the holistic transition from recovery focused care to end of life care. Dr. Porock calls this transition "recognizing dying." She recorded a TEDx talk on this topic called Healthy Dying.

Dr. Porock has collaborated with interdisciplinary research teams to refine and investigate the care of people with dementia in long-term care facilities and hospitals. She has focused on the application of person centered care for dementia patients. Dr. Porock established the University of Buffalo Institute for Person Centered Care (IPCC) in

2012. The John R. Oishei Foundation and the Office of Research and Economic Development of the University of Buffalo funded the institute for three years.

INTERVIEW

Jean Galiana (JG): Can you tell me about your career path and what led you to conduct research with a focus on dementia care?

Davina Porock (DP): I worked mainly in oncology when I was an active clinical nurse. I found that much of my work was in palliative care. I decided to go back to school for my master's degree. I conducted my first research project during that process. As I continued working in clinical nursing, I realized that I really wanted to do research more than anything else.

I shifted gears and received a teaching position at one of the local universities in Perth, West Australia. While I was a clinical teacher, I started my PhD with a focus in radiation oncology. Radiation oncology was an expedient topic at the time. My career focus became clear after I received my PhD and shifted into gerontology oncology.

Through my work in gerontology oncology, I became fascinated with trying to improve end of life care rather than focusing only on curing cancer. It became clear to me that any patient who has cancer has a better chance of receiving palliative or hospice care than an older person who doesn't have cancer. It was very difficult to receive palliative and hospice support for seniors when I began my career in gerontology oncology.

I combined my research career with my love of travel. I have worked in Australia, the United Kingdom, and the United States. I have also been a visiting professor in Malaysia and India.

While in the United Kingdom, I worked at the University of Nottingham and was a member of a large multidisciplinary gerontology research group.

There, the National Institute for Health Research supported our work with a large five-year program grant. The National Institute for Health Research is the UK equivalent of the National Institutes of Health in the US. One of our programs dealt with older adults with dementia in the hospital setting.

In the mid-2000s, I began focusing on end of life care for older adults with dementia. We developed a specialist unit in the hospital for people with dementia who were hospitalized for common issues that could not be controlled outside of the hospital. These patients were in the hospital for the usual challenges that send older people to the hospital, except they also had dementia. We designed a specialist unit for this cohort and performed trial tests. While developing the new unit, I trained in person centered care at the University of Bradford, and introduced person centered care to the operations of the specialist unit.

I moved to the University at Buffalo in 2010 and was there for five years. During that time, I had the opportunity to focus on person centeredness and was able to establish the Institute for Person Centered Care. I am currently the vice provost for Academic Personnel at Lehman College, City University of New York, in the Bronx.

JG: What are the biggest accomplishments of the Institute for Person Centered Care?

DP: For my research, we examined how to measure person centeredness—how to determine person centered care is happening. We also studied stress levels as a way to understand how person centered care works from a physiological perspective as well as psychosocial.

People used to say, "Oh, it is just about being nice. If everyone is just nice to the elderly people, we'll be fine." It is much more than that. Patient centeredness is not the classic picture of old people parked around the edge of the nursing home lounge, asleep in their chairs. The practice of only keeping residents clean and dry actually does more harm than good.

People with more advanced dementia can have what are sometimes called "difficult behaviors." They can be aggressive. Sometimes they might hit, bite, or scream. People with advanced dementia can become agitated and pace the floor, trying to escape, or repeatedly call out. These behaviors are misunderstood.

Someone with dementia cannot comprehend what or who is coming at him or her. Someone with dementia cannot comprehend people talking or doing things quickly. The only thing they can do to take back control is to stop, hit, or resist in other ways. These behaviors need to be understood as stress reactions, not bad behavior. We have created a malignant social environment that does not treat these behaviors as distressed responses. Dementia patients have few other options than to respond negatively. Dementia patients want to have control over their environments and what happens to them, just like any other person.

We can reduce their stress by changing to a person centered approach. For example, we can change the way we speak to people. We can ensure that we do not take people by surprise. We can give visual cues such as hand cues to say what we are doing instead of only verbal cues. A specific example is to take the hand of the patient and help them clean their teeth rather than brushing their teeth for them. These changes are very simple things, but they all take time. People have to be reminded that these person centered approaches are important.

The challenge is how to apply the person centered care

processes in institutional settings. It can be difficult to get traditional nursing homes to include the values, likes, and dislikes of the individuals in their care model. Nursing homes are set up like hospitals. I have conducted a very small study where I took saliva samples to measure the stress hormone cortisol from the residents with dementia in a large dementia unit. I am still analyzing that data.

JG: I noticed you have several published studies dealing with dementia care in long-term skilled nursing facilities and hospitals. Is there anything from that research that you would like to share?

DP: I think hospital and long-term care facility employees often think person centered care requires taking the time to build a relationship with the dementia patient and their family. In the hospital, people say, "I do not have time for that," and they honestly do not. However, it is possible to find a workaround to understand what helps a person feel settled as quickly as possible. If a patient gets very agitated, what is the best way to help soothe and calm her?

To address this, we developed a document called About Me. We asked the family member, nursing home aide, or whoever brought the person into the hospital to fill it out. This document is used to share personal details, like the important people, pets, or things that the person likes to talk about. What soothes them? What agitates them? What do they enjoy? What work did they used to do? This enables caregivers to engage dementia patients in meaningful conversations. This is an expedient method to build a patient centered relationship that would usually develop naturally over a longer period of time.

We also changed visiting hours and asked the relatives to come in and help so that the patients could interact with familiar people. Additionally, we made sure that as soon as the seniors were physically well enough, they had to get up and get dressed so they would not forget how. Losing skills is one of the biggest problems of hospitalization for people living with dementia. If you keep doing the basic activities of daily living, you are less likely to lose them.

Another issue in dementia care in the acute care setting is moving or relocating people. When someone with dementia or delirium along with dementia goes to the hospital because of a fall, for example, they are moved around quite a bit. They have a fall, which is already disorientating, and then they go into the stressful setting of an ambulance. Next, they get to the emergency room and are often moved to some sort of assessment area while they wait for a bed. Then they go up to the actual nursing floor. Afterward, they might even get moved around that floor.

Every time you change the place or the people who are interacting with a person who has dementia, disorientation and fear increase. Staffing consistency and minimizing change can reduce distress and disorientation. We need standardized models of care that address changing caregivers and locations for dementia patients.

People with dementia are not good historians. They often cannot remember to tell their relative or clinician what it was that happened to them. Most professionals are not well educated about dementia and delirium. Not at all. That needs to change, given the rise in the senior population and the accompanying increased rates of dementia and delirium. Staff must make a point of telling the family what is happening and confirming the accuracy of the information given by the patient.

The hospitals in the UK generally have shared bathrooms. They do not have private rooms like they do in America. The bathrooms were all beautifully clean with white tiles, white walls, and a white toilet. If a patient has visual spatial problems associated with dementia and everything in a room is white, he or she will not actually be able to see exactly where the toilet is. This results in patients missing the toilet and ending up half on and half off or on the floor. One of the best things we ever did was simply putting black toilet seats on all of the toilets.

Signage adjustment can be valuable in caring for patients with dementia. We put in very clear signs with black writing on a yellow background. This is the last combination that can be recognized by someone with visual problems. We also moved the signs to eye level so people did not have to search for them. Patients with dementia recognize the older, universal signs long into their disease because they are embedded in old memory.

When people with dementia pace, they may be feeling that they are trying to get somewhere or find someone. When they are unsuccessful, it can cause agitation. They do not necessarily forget that they have been back and forth in the same place, but they know they haven't found what they wanted. They know it, and it is annoying. They have the emotion even if they cannot remember or articulate what caused it.

We had a long ward so we put electronic pictures at each end. On one end, we had a picture of Nottingham from the old days that would give the staff something to talk about with patients. On the other end, the picture was something different, like a field of flowers. The pictures changed electronically so that there was always something new and stimulating to look at. None of this was terribly expensive.

One of the more expensive changes we made was adding additional staff. We added people in occupational therapy, physical therapy, and people to support activities so there was always something going on for the patients. We also got the patients up and out of bed as much as possible. We brought people to the table together to eat instead of letting them eat alone in bed. This kept the patients up and doing normal things even when they were in the hospital.

The length of stay for a dementia patient hospitalized with another illness was typically longer than those hospitalized with the same illness who did not have dementia. We were able to reduce the length of stay for the dementia patient to equal those without dementia. We also saw the days at home post discharge decrease significantly.

JG: Were you able to replicate that model anywhere else?

DP: I have tied the model to my teaching. I have not replicated the specialist unit anywhere. I believe some places in the UK have.

JG: In a recent publication, you surveyed dementia patients and caregivers of dementia patients to determine their priorities for research and public policy spending. What inspired you to do that research? What were your findings?

DP: The National Alzheimer's Plan Act (NAPA) is the national dementia plan of the US. Every other country names its national program the National Dementia Plan, but in the United States it is named the National Alzheimer's Plan, hence my irritation about people mixing up dementia and Alzheimer's. One is exclusive and the other is inclusive. Dementia is the inclusive term. In fact, the Alzheimer's Association will say Alzheimer's and related dementias when it should be dementia or dementia including Alzheimer's. I am not saying that they have not done good work. The Alzheimer's organizations have done great work. I just wish that the emphasis was not only on one disease.

The National Alzheimer's Plan Act council meets every quarter to oversee the workings of the Act, including funding support. Four out of the five goals that are published on their website are about care, but the vast majority of their funding goes to research. The research only includes basic science and drug development. I want that research to continue, but there are many people who are managing dementia day to day. They are incurring a huge financial burden with very limited networks within society and the healthcare system to support them. Like every other chronic illness, dementia affects the whole family, not just the person with the condition.

JG: Are you are suggesting a reprioritization of funding?

DP: Yes. We need systems in place that will always be in place for everyone thereafter. Yes, the research will go on, but there is very little in place to support people living with dementia and their caregivers. We have established networks to support people with breast cancer, prostate cancer, and many other kinds of cancer, including childhood cancer. The support networks and fundraisers, among other things, are ingrained in our systems. We need a government funded priority that creates a coordinated approach to provision of services, education and training, stigma reduction, and services and support for dementia.

The disparity of the National Alzheimer's Plan Act funding is huge: One hundred million dollars a year goes to basic science and drug development. Ten million a year goes to programs to support the care of people with Alzheimer's disease. It is an incredible disparity. The shame is compounded when we know the drug companies will not give us a discount on the drugs that they eventually do develop, despite the government funding of the drug development. In fact, the medicines cost more in the United States than anywhere else in the world.

JG: Do funding priorities need to change?

DP: Yes, they do. One of the most important aspects of the growth of dementia diagnoses is that the highest growth rates will be in the low and middle income countries, not in the United States and countries with older populations like the United Kingdom and Europe. People are living longer in the low and middle income countries because their economies are developing. Healthcare, nutrition, and clean water are improving. Western medicine helps them to live longer with heart disease or cancer, which enables them to live long enough to develop dementia.

Once appropriate care systems are developed, there will be a plan for everyone thereafter. Yes, the basic science needs to be done, and drug development and other treatments need to be done. It is going to be decades, if ever, before we find cures. Then there will be other illnesses. So far, no one has lived forever.

One of the painful stigmas of having dementia, particularly in the earliest stages, is that people automatically assume you have suddenly become stupid. There are some great people who publicly demonstrate that this is not the case. A perfect example is Michael Ellenbogen. He has had Alzheimer's for more than ten years. He is still an active advocate. He continues to advocate at National Alzheimer's Plan Act meetings. He also wrote an eBook entitled *From Corner Office to Alzheimer's*. He continues to write blog posts. People think he does not have dementia. He does. His mission is to make a difference in public understanding and demonstrate that it is possible to live well with dementia.

JG: I really enjoyed your TEDx talk on Healthy Dying. Can you talk about your concept of healthy dying?

DP: My concept of healthy dying is that dying, going from being alive to being dead, is a transition like any other transition we have in our lives. Every transition we make has a physiological, psychological, and social element to it. We recognize and even celebrate them. Being born is the first one. We go from being a fetus to becoming an infant. This transition is the birthing process. Later, we go from childhood to adolescence to adulthood. Even socially constructed transitions like retiring or adopting have physiological responses. These transitions are very important. They are all developmental.

Death is the same. The transition is dying. What is going on physiologically? What is going on psychologically? What is going on sociologically? Why do we treat it differently from the other transitions? Why don't we recognize dying for what it is, instead of looking to healthcare?

Healthcare helps a person live longer, healthier lives. Healthcare is about prolonging life. Dying care is not about prolonging life. It is about being with the person as they die and making it as comfortable and as good as possible. Often we do not stop giving healthcare. That is the problem. We keep sticking people with needles. We keep thinking that we can fix them or arrest the process. This is not person centered. It is medicine and system centered. It is not about the person who is dying or their family. We need to stop providing health-care for someone who is dying and instead switch to dying care. The crux of the problem is knowing that you are going to die and having that conversation about what you want.

The palliative care movement is about making a good death by honoring what the patient finds important in his or her last phase. Palliative care professionals and geriatricians are the two specialties most different from the other medical specialties because they are not focused on one disease. They are focused on the whole person and their family. Their ideas about the importance of living and dying well are different. I ended that TEDx talk with a quote from Erik Erikson, the developmental psychologist, who said, "The best thing a parent can do for their child is not be frightened of dying."

JG: Do you think end of life conversations and planning should be part of the primary care doctor's protocol?

DP: Yes, I do, but there would likely be resistance to that. I think advanced care planning is essential for all of us to do. I think we should start writing out advanced care plans when we are young and modify as we learn and grow wiser. University education should include death and dying education. We are creating the most educated people in our society, but we do not talk about the one thing that will happen to every single person.

JG: Did you experience that in nursing school?

DP: There is some education around dying, but the emphasis is wrong. It is out of balance. We spent a lot of time in nursing school talking about fetal development. There is only a very small proportion of nurses who actually deal with fetal development in their professional practice.

I have taught many classes on the care of the dying. I ask my graduate students who have been practicing nurses, "How many of you have actually delivered a baby, not counting the personal delivery of your own children or watching your wife have a baby? How many as a professional nurse have delivered a baby?" In a class of about thirty, one or two students will raise their hands. Then I ask, "How many of you have sat with someone who was dying?" Two hands, two legs, and all of their fingers go up because it is countless.

In education, we do not spend enough time talking about aging, disability, and the dying process. Student nurses will be able to tell you about the stages of labor. Even in the National Council License Exam, which is the licensing exam for nurses, they will ask questions about caring for someone in labor. There is not the same emphasis in the curriculum or in the National Council License Exam on the care of someone who is dying and their family.

When I was a student midwife, a tutor came in and said, "There is a woman next door in labor, and there is absolutely no one with her. She is full term, and there is no husband, no mother, no obstetrician, and no midwife in her room. What is going to happen? You have twenty minutes to write down what is going to happen." We came up with multiple disasters. The tutor then said, "No, she is going to have a baby. That is what is going to happen." This poses a few questions: Why do you need to be there? What is it a midwife brings to the delivery process? If you left her alone, she would still have a baby.

When I decided not to be a midwife, I realized that I found the old, sick, and dying patients to be much more interesting. Now I say to my students, after telling the midwifery story, "There is a person in the next room dying and there is nobody with them. There is no spouse, no children, no doctor, no nurse, no one. What is going to happen?"

The students know the answer and say, "The person is going to die." "Can you change that outcome?" They answer, "No."

Then I ask the same question, "Why do we need to be there?" The dying do not need healthcare anymore, but they do need dying care. They need someone to give them comfort and security. As someone once wisely said, "An unaccompanied death is uncivilized."

JG: Do you have any research plans for the future?

DP: I have what I call "the spit study," which is the saliva study I mentioned for dementia care mapping. I have a lot of data that needs to be published. I am also working with a colleague at the University of Buffalo, Dr. Yu-Ping Chang, who is an exceptional gerontology nurse researcher and a statistician. She and I are beginning to collect New York State nursing home data to study person centered nursing. Person centered care is now mandated. We want to determine how we can grade the level of implementation of person centered care. We plan to compare all of the levels of care with resident and organizational outcomes.

Much of the information we are collecting is from the Minimum Data Set. Every nursing home that gets paid by

Medicare or Medicaid must complete the Minimum Data Set quarterly for each resident. It is a huge dataset owned by the government. Dr. Yu-Ping Chang and I did this study in one nursing home that is published in the Journal of American Medical Directors Association. We are planning to repeat that study for the entire state.

JG: That sounds exciting.

DP: It keeps me out of mischief.

JG: Thank you for your time and a most interesting discussion.

— END OF INTERVIEW —

A Palliative Approach to Dementia Care

An interview with **Lotta Roupe**

Introduction

In 1996, Queen Silvia of Sweden founded Stiftelsen Silviahemmet (Silviahemmet), a foundation that provides a day care center and education in dementia care. The aim of Stiftelsen Silviahemmet is to provide the highest possible standard of living for individuals who suffer from dementia and for their relatives. The Silvia Sister education program is named after Queen Silvia and is based on a palliative care philosophy that includes four central aspects of dementia care.

The first aspect of the palliative care philosophy, control of symptoms and person centered care, involves active prevention and a focus on reducing the symptoms of dementia. The second aspect, communication and relations, addresses the importance of caregivers taking time to know the person who suffers from dementia and to create a relationship with the individual. The third aspect emphasizes the need for teamwork among caregivers and includes a focus on learning from each other about how best to deliver dementia care. The fourth aspect, support for relatives, strengthens the role of relatives and ensures that relatives achieve the highest possible life quality.

After a hiatus, Silviahemmet relaunched the Silvia Sister dementia education program in 2004, in cooperation with Sophiahemmet University College. Sophiahemmet University College is an institution of higher education for nurses and assistant nurses. The Silvia Sister course is provided online. The course provides sixty university credits. Students must be an assistant nurse or higher to qualify for the program. After graduation, participants receive the title Silvia Sister from Queen Silvia.

Silviahemmet certifies homecare organizations and delivers courses for relatives. The director of Silviahemmet, Wilhelmina Hoffman, is also the director of the Swedish Dementia Center. The role of the Swedish Dementia Center is to spread knowledge about dementia through online courses.

In this interview, Lotta Roupe, an assistant nurse, Silvia Sister, and manager of the day care center of Silviahemmet, talks about the history of Silviahemmet and its palliative care philosophy. Ms. Roupe also gives an overview of the day care center and the different courses and certifications offered by Stiftelsen Silviahemmet.

About Lotta Roupe

Lotta Roupe holds a degree in assistant nursing. Since 1976, she has worked as an assistant nurse in elderly care at group homes, for homecare services, and at nursing homes in Sweden. In 2001, she graduated from the one-year education program at Stiftelsen Silviahemmet and received the title Silvia Sister. In 2002, she started to work as a Silvia Sister at Silviahemmet in Stockholm. At Silviahemmet, her main responsibility is as manager of the day care center. Ms. Roupe also teaches courses in dementia care and manages reflection sessions.

INTERVIEW

Sofia Widén (SW): Please describe the background of the day care center at Stiftelsen Silviahemmet (Silviahemmet).

Lotta Roupe (LR): Stiftelsen Silviahemmet started as a dementia care school for assistant nurses. The school invited people who suffer from dementia to spend their days at the day care center. The daily residents provided clinical experience to the assistant nurses. Over the years, Silviahemmet developed into a permanent day care center. The purpose remains the same: to spread knowledge about dementia care to improve quality of life and to provide education in the palliative care philosophy.

Silviahemmet has about eight to ten visitors every day. Silviahemmet currently serves about eighteen people, which corresponds to about one hundred seventy daily visits per month. Individuals visit the day care center up to five times a week. The day care center delivers person centered dementia care. This means that the individual, the visitor, is always the highest priority for the staff members. The work starts with an extensive review of the needs of the visitors. The schedule of activities is flexible. If visitors want to go for a walk or a run or go to the gym, the staff member will adjust. After all, the person who suffers from dementia knows best what he or she needs. There is a clear structure in the work at the day care center. This structure is also flexible and provides room for creativity and flexibility.

SW: How do you enroll at Silviahemmet?

LR: Silviahemmet is a foundation. This means that individuals either pay out of pocket or receive funding from the local municipality through a support agent system. Most people apply for funding from their municipality. We care for many younger elderly at Silviahemmet. These younger individuals are between sixty to sixty-five years of age. At the age of sixty-five, you have the right to elder care. The problem is that most people who visit dementia day care centers in Sweden are older than sixty-five. People who are sixty-five often feel very young around people aged eighty or older. At Silviahemmet, we offer two days reserved for the young elderly, while three days are set for mixed ages.

SW: How much does it cost to enroll for care at Silviahemmet?

LR: A visit to Silviahemmet costs around one thousand Swedish kronor (around 125 US dollars) per day. This is a competitive price compared to what other day care centers charge, but the price does not cover all costs. We also receive grants and revenues from our courses and certifications.

SW: Which types of care providers can obtain a Stiftelsen Silviahemmet certification?

LR: Care homes and day care centers can obtain certification from Silviahemmet. The certification indicates the level of knowledge of the care provider. The certification process is for anyone who works at a day care center or in a care home. Anyone from the janitor to the highest managers can complete a three-day training in dementia care. The course covers aspects such as different dementia illnesses, changes in the brain, symptoms of dementia, and care strategies.

The second stage in the certification process is to choose work leaders. The work leaders participate in an additional one-day training in dementia care. The work leaders supervise the care home employees to make sure that the employees follow the Silviahemmet care philosophy.

The third stage of the certification process is to send two nurses for a three-day training session to become reflection leaders. We hold the training either at Silviahemmet or at the care home. The reflection leaders lead monthly sessions for employees at the care home. The session lasts between one and two hours, with the purpose of reflecting on the dementia care provided and potential improvements.

If a care home provider becomes certified at Silviahemmet, the certification is valid for three years. We evaluate the certificate after one and a half years to ensure that the care home provider is upholding the required standards. During the certification process, all participants take a test. If the total test score of the care home is above seventy percent, the home receives the certificate. The advantage of the certification is that each individual feels strengthened in his or her role as a caregiver. As a result, each person feels more confident in his or her care approach and residents obtain better care. We can deliver each course at Silviahemmet in Stockholm or at the care home, whether that is in Sweden or abroad.

SW: Can you give an example of a work leader?

LR: A work leader could be a director or a nurse who is responsible for a department or unit. Some care providers also have assistant nurses as team leaders. A team leader has a similar function as a work leader and can attend the second stage in the certification process.

SW: Who receives the certification, the individuals or the care provider?

LR: The care provider receives the certification, not the individuals. The individuals receive a course certificate. A Silvia Sister is a person who is graduated from the Sophiahemmet University College. There is an important distinction between a Silvia Sister who graduated from the college and an individual who receives the course certificate from Silviahemmet.

SW: Do you evaluate your certification? What is the reaction from the participants?

LR: No. We do not evaluate our certification, but I have heard positive reactions from the participants as well as from the leaders of their care units. The participants feel more confident in their roles. They collaborate better with each other. The participants are also more likely to ask for help and are more secure in their image and attitude toward both visitors and relatives.

SW: Does the staff of Silviahemmet also work with the certification?

LR: Yes. I do part time education and certification, and my colleague Eva Jönsson works full time with education and certification. We also receive external help from Silvia Sisters connected to us.

SW: Do you certify international care providers?

LR: Yes. We invite international visitors to Silviahemmet. We also visit care providers abroad. I went to visit the Order of Malta in Germany last week. Representatives from the Order of Malta have also visited us for an instructor's course. The course was a one-week intensive training for instructors to learn about the palliative care philosophy of Silviahemmet. The content was more thorough than our basic courses. The instructors also learned how to convey the care philosophy to other staff members at their care homes.

SW: What type of other courses do you offer?

LR: We offer a range of courses, from shorter basic courses to longer medical training. The courses are either held at Silviahemmet, at Sophiahemmet University College, at the Karolinska Institute, or at an external care provider.

In 2008, Sophiahemmet University College and Silviahemmet launched a degree program for nurses in dementia care. This is a one-year web based distance learning program at half speed that provides thirty university credits. Four years later, we launched the first Silvia Doctor education program with the Karolinska Institute. This is a two-year web based program that grants a master's degree in dementia care. Currently, twenty-five doctors are participating in the course. In November, the Karolinska Institute and Silviahemmet launched a master's degree program for physical therapists and occupational therapists. This is also offered online.

SW: Can you tell me about your palliative care philosophy?

LR: The palliative care philosophy of Silviahemmet is based on four key components. The objective of the care philosophy is to provide the highest possible quality of life for individuals who suffer from dementia and for their families.

The first component is control of symptoms and person centered care. This component involves active prevention and a focus on reducing the symptoms of dementia. If an individual starts looking for the bathroom and cannot find it, a staff member may intervene early to guide that person to the bathroom. This intervention prevents that person from feeling confused, anxious, or frustrated because he or she cannot find the bathroom.

The role of caring for people who suffer from dementia involves knowing the person, being able to read signals, being able to step in and provide a hand of support, but also being able to reflect carefully upon when to intervene and when to step back. There are many different illnesses involved in dementia, and there are equally as many symptoms. Some people lose their sense of orientation. Others struggle to express themselves. The role of the caregiver is to understand each individual and work around his or her symptoms.

The second component of the palliative care philosophy is communication and relations. To deliver person centered dementia care, every caregiver needs to take the time to get to know the person who suffers from dementia. Caregivers need to create a relationship with the individual to deliver person centered care. Caregivers do this by spending time with the individual and talking about what matters to him or her. The caregivers eat together and sit down to have coffee with the visitors. It is also important to create trust. A person who suffers from dementia must trust you.

The palliative care philosophy recognizes no "us and them" divide. The staff members are not viewed as caregivers, and they do not view themselves as caregivers. The staff members view themselves as friends of the visitors and communicate in that way. This is an important element of the care philosophy, especially for the younger elderly who suffer from dementia. The younger elderly do not want to be treated like patients. The younger elderly want to participate in activities and enjoy company during the day. The younger elderly need support but want to feel normal.

The third component of the palliative care philosophy is teamwork among the caregivers. Caregivers need to create relationships with each other to learn more about how to deliver dementia care in the best way. Caregivers need to talk to each other and build relationships with other team members at the care facility. Caregivers also need to create relationships with important people in the visitors' lives, such as relatives, homecare workers, and other healthcare professionals. Caregivers need to understand that teamwork is a critical aspect of dementia care and that their team is larger than their colleagues at the care home.

The fourth and last component is to provide support for relatives. Silviahemmet invites family members to the care home, educates them, and makes sure that the wishes of family members are heard. If relatives want to be actively involved and learn about what their loved ones are doing at the day care center, then the staff members brief the relatives on a daily basis. If relatives prefer to have less intensive contact with the staff, then their wishes are respected. The staff members keep a journal to make sure that they touch base with relatives at least once a month. We communicate with relatives over the phone or via text messages, emails, or other avenues. Silviahemmet strengthens the role of relatives and ensures that relatives can achieve the highest possible quality of life as well. This is a critical element in the palliative care philosophy.

SW: How do you ensure the quality of care at Silviahemmet?

LR: Every six months, we reevaluate each person's care plan and how well it is meeting the four components of the palliative care philosophy. We individualize these care plans for each individual. The care plans also serve as documentation for the local municipalities. In the care plans, the caregiver describes a range of activities an individual may like. Over time, we revise the care plan to suit the capabilities of each individual. For example, one guest may be able to take long walks and paint in the beginning of his or her visits to the day care center. After about six months, the dementia may have caused certain physical and cognitive functions to deteriorate. That individual may no longer be able to paint or take long walks. That is why the staff members continuously update and revise the care plans. Every six months, we revise each component of the care philosophy to suit the individual and his or her needs. At the same time, we hold a continuous dialogue with the individual's relatives, since the relatives may also change their minds when the needs of the individual change.

SW: What is included in the courses you provide to relatives? Are they as intensive as the courses you offer to care providers?

LR: No, not really. The education for relatives is a one-day course that begins to cover the brain, dementia diseases, and symptoms of dementia. During the afternoon, the relatives learn how to communicate with an individual who suffers from dementia and about the experiences of others caring for loved ones with dementia. The education for relatives involves a large component in which relatives share their experiences of caring for someone with dementia. I cannot tell the relatives what it is like to live with someone who suffers from dementia. Instead, relatives teach us what it is like to live with someone who suffers from dementia. Relatives need to exchange ideas and experiences. That is how we can support relatives.

SW: In the future, how will Silviahemmet continue to develop? Are there any changes coming?

LR: We will continue with the day care center and our courses will be held at Silviahemmet, in other parts of Sweden, and abroad. We try to plan and develop the day care center along with our visitors and evaluate our work every day after closing hours.

SW: Do you think the world will be able to take care of all individuals who suffer from dementia and offer them high quality dementia care?

LR: Yes. I am hopeful for the future. Today, people arrive from all over the world to Sweden. They bring with them their culture and respect for the elderly. Swedish people must learn from other cultures how to respect older people and behave with dignity. We have the knowledge to make a change, but we also need the necessary resources. I believe the future lies in flexibility, both in resources and in the approach to dementia care.

SW: Thank you, Lotta, for an interesting interview.

LR: Thank you, Sofia.

— END OF INTERVIEW —

Person Directed Dementia Living

An interview with **Beatitudes Campus**

Background

Beatitudes Campus is a life plan community in Phoenix, Arizona. The twenty-five acre campus is home to seven hundred residents. The campus has a host of amenities including a fitness studio, a swimming pool, a library, numerous restaurants ranging from coffee shop to bistro to fine dining, and even a lovely bar. The restaurants and bar are open to the public and are used frequently.

Other amenities on the campus include a hair salon, a bank, a chapel, arts and crafts and ceramics studios, a woodworking shop, garden areas, and walking paths. There is a doctor and a medical staff on campus. Museum quality art can be seen throughout the community. There are over ninety clubs at Beatitudes, all founded and run by the residents.

Beatitudes Campus has been conducting research into person directed dementia living for decades. Researchers at Beatitudes Campus have designed an evidence based model for dementia care called Comfort Matters, a model that has been introduced to thousands of long-term care staff, medical providers, and students throughout the world. Through the two-year training program of Tena Alonzo, Karen Mitchell, and their team, the Comfort Matters concepts have been replicated in long-term care organizations throughout the United States.

In this interview, Tena Alonzo, Karen Mitchell, and Ivan Hilton give examples of person directed living and share how they transformed the Beatitudes Campus into a fully person directed facility. They detail the philosophies and values of the Comfort Matters model and how the model was successfully operationalized, even in their late stage dementia residence, Vermilion Cliffs.

About Karen Mitchell

Karen Mitchell, RN, BSN. Educator of Comfort Matters.

Karen Mitchell has spent the past four decades improving the quality of life for older adults and their families in the long-term care setting. Throughout her career, Ms. Mitchell has served in a variety of roles including nursing assistant, charge nurse, nursing instructor, nursing supervisor, assistant director, and director of nursing. Karen joined the staff at Beatitudes Campus in 1983 and has since been a driving force in developing and implementing evidence based, best practice care. Her work has been published in the *New York Times*, the *New Yorker Magazine*, and the *Journal of Hospice and Palliative Nursing*. Ms. Mitchell received her Registered Nursing degree from Maria College in Albany, New York, in 1975 and a Bachelor of Science in Nursing from the University of Phoenix in 1989.

About Tena Alonzo

Tena R. M. Alonzo, MA. Director of Education and Research.
Director of Comfort Matters.

Ms. Alonzo is the director of education and research and the director of Comfort Matters at Beatitudes Campus in Phoenix, Arizona. She is also the education director for Palliative Care for the Advanced Dementia Training and Implementation Project in New York City in collaboration with Caring Kind (formerly the Alzheimer's Association New York City Chapter). She currently serves as a technical expert for the Initiative to Improve Dementia Care and Reduce Antipsychotic Medication for the Centers for Medicare and Medicaid.

Tena Alonzo's research focuses on developing comfort focused best practice for addressing dementia related behavior; decreasing antipsychotic, anxiolytic, and sedative medications; enhancing pain management; eliminating physical restraints; preventing rejection of care; understanding behavior as a method of communication; addressing dining and nutrition concerns; enhancing fall reduction techniques; and educating caregiving staff in understanding the progression of dementia.

Ms. Alonzo's work has been published in more than twenty-five books and scholarly journals. Ms. Alonzo speaks nationally and internationally as a keynote speaker, featured speaker, panel member, and facilitator on evidence based, caregiving practices for people with dementia.

Ms. Alonzo earned a Bachelor of Science in Psychology and Biology in 1983 and a Master of Administration in Theoretical Psychology in 1985 from Northern Arizona University. She is currently pursuing a doctoral degree in biomedical ethics.

About Ivan Hilton

Ivan Hilton, MA, FACHE. Director of Business Development for Comfort Matters.

Ivan Hilton has more than forty years of experience in the development and implementation of best practices in acute healthcare settings. He has held a variety of roles including microbiologist, assistant hospital administrator, business developer, and consultant. Most recently, in an acute healthcare setting, he served as vice president of ancillary and clinical support services for the John C. Lincoln Health Network located in Phoenix, Arizona.

Mr. Hilton has a Bachelor of Science degree in Medical Technology from the University of Utah and a master's degree in Hospital Administration from Central Michigan University. He is board certified in healthcare management and is a Fellow in the American College of Healthcare Executives.

INTERVIEW

Jean Galiana (JG): What drew you to the long-term care industry?

Karen Mitchell (KM): My grandmother. People are usually drawn to elder care because of a family member. My grandmother emigrated from England. Her father worked in a cigar factory. She was one of nine children. We lived in adjoining apartments. She was on the bottom flat and we were on the top flat. She was a nursing assistant in an oncology unit at a hospital in Albany, New York. When she became ill, she was not dying quickly enough in the hospital so they told her that she had to move to a nursing home. Because she had seen the deplorable conditions in nursing homes back then, she was frightened about the prospect of living in a nursing home. This was in the 1960s, when nursing homes were scary places. She was terrified. She died before they were able to move her. That experience set my resolve to help create better care options for the other grandmothers.

Tena Alonzo (TA): My grandmother was diagnosed with early onset Alzheimer's around 1982. She was not yet sixty. It was the first time I had ever heard the term Alzheimer's. I was an undergraduate studying psychology and biology. I was planning to be a professor. From her diagnosis to her death was approximately eighteen months. Generally early onset Alzheimer's progresses more quickly, which is a blessing in some ways. I saw good aspects and bad aspects of healthcare during her experience with Alzheimer's disease. At the time of her death, I decided to be part of a team that enhances the quality of life for people with dementia. I changed direction and attained my master's in geropsychology. I spent the early part of my career in geropsychology trying to improve the quality of life for older people with dementia and other chronic mental illnesses. It was difficult to witness the way the care providers were treating people with dementia and mental illness. The individuals had their sense of autonomy undermined. The people with schizophrenia would receive more attention and more support than the person who had issues related specifically to Alzheimer's disease.

JG: By attention and support, do you mean medically or psychologically?

TA: Both. Those living with dementia were placed on the bottom of the priority list. It was a terrible situation for those who had dementia and mental illness such as a history of schizophrenia, schizoaffective disorder, and bipolar disorder.

Approximately twelve years into my career, I realized that I was in the wrong place to make the level of impact that I had envisioned. If I wanted to effect change I needed to be part of another system. My colleague, Jill Hamilton, who was the medical director here until recently, asked me to join the team at Beatitudes. When I arrived, it was clear that we had a good team comprised of people who cared about the residents. We struggled to develop the culture, policies, and procedures to become as radically person centered as we are today. I knew that we did not know everything we needed to know about serving those living with dementia. I began the journey of research and discovery. We wanted to learn what a completely person directed model of care looked like in action.

Initially we had a traditional model of care with a strong medical component. We had a wonderful clinical director, Dr. Gary Martin, who is a great geropsychologist, and Jill Hamilton as our medical director. She is an internist and a board certified geriatrician and palliative care provider. We had a good, but traditional team. We knew how to administer medicine and treat medical issues, but we were not yet caring for the whole person. In essence, a traditional model of care without the other components is hospital care. They send you into a hospital, fix your problem, and send you home. You endure some of the distress and upset associated with the short stay situation because they are going to make you better. They want to cure you as quickly as possible to get you back to your life. There is no quick fix or cure for dementia. This is long-term living. No one is going home. We needed to progress beyond being solely focused on the medical to include the mind and the spirit.

JG: How did you begin progressing to include the mind and the spirit?

TA: We began to overlay a social model on top of the medical model. We discovered along the way that we did not know very much about taking care of people with dementia. That was not our fault. No one knew much about caring for people living with dementia twenty years ago. Today, many still do not understand the culture needed to create person centered dementia care.

JG: Did the board support your efforts to learn a new care model and implement a new organizational culture?

TA: We had support from the top management down to nearly everyone else. Beatitudes Campus is an organization that was founded on faith and is driven by innovation. The leaders of the Beatitudes organization have historically embraced a strong sense of social justice. We are affiliated with the United Church of Christ, also called the Beatitudes Church, which supports social justice for all people.

JG: What is the history of Beatitudes Campus?

TA: Reverend Dr. Culver, the first pastor of the Church of Beatitudes, which is just down the street, was visiting one of his parishioners in a nursing home. He witnessed deplorable conditions and was encouraged by his wife to meet with the congregation to determine whether they could help. He rallied the church to create the Beatitudes Campus in the early 1960s. Many parishioners mortgaged their homes to contribute financially. The pastor and other church leaders chose to cancel plans to build their sanctuary and to contribute those funds to building Beatitudes Campus instead. Reverend Dr. Culver believed that older adults needed a place where they could live, learn, and grow every day of their lives. He lives on the campus now. His vision and mission established our foundation of innovation. Years later, our organizational culture of innovation enabled us to develop the Comfort Matters evidence based training.

KM: We hold that history and their commitment close to our hearts. We are determined to continue their mission.

JG: Did the church members volunteer to spend time with the Beatitudes residents?

TA: Yes, and they still do today. Advocacy and social justice are fundamental principles of the Beatitudes Campus because of our roots in the United Church of Christ. We began our exploration from those commitments and beliefs. We are dedicated to creating a community that is inclusive for our diverse residents. We strive to create a place of comfort for people who have trouble thinking, because they deserve a home as well. It was a labor of love for everyone involved. We knew we could design a new model of dementia care that was more person centered than anyone had yet conceived of. We did not know what the model would be, but we knew it would be different. Fortunately, there were not many egos in our way. The purity of our desire to make life better for those living with dementia made Comfort Matters possible.

JG: Do the Vermilion Cliffs memory residents have their own rooms?

Ivan Hilton (IH): We have single and double occupancy rooms. The double rooms are large. They were built to house three. The residents bring their own furnishings and decorations. We find ways to arrange the furnishings to create a fair level of privacy. If roommates are not happy living with each other, we find roommates who are a better match.

The new center that we are planning will have private rooms only. The structure will be based on the small home model. It will be a multi-story building with safe balconies for residents to experience fresh air and sunshine. We will also include places for safe wandering.

JG: How many rooms are you planning to build in the new structure?

TA: The need for memory living residences is great here in Phoenix. We could fill Vermilion Cliffs many times over today if we had the space. We are grappling with meeting the great need in our community and creating the small home environment that can house many. The average age of our seven hundred and twenty residents is eighty-seven. Many will likely need memory residences.

JG: What are your thoughts regarding the built environment?

IH: Architecture is not critical to provide comfort for people. We are a perfect example. We will not go into organizations where we are conducting our two-year training and demand that they build green houses or small homes. We do believe the built environment can help to support the care culture, but it is not imperative.

TA: We want environment to match program. That is one of the reasons we are preparing to build new residences.

JG: What percentage of your residents pay privately verses publicly?

TA: Sixty percent of our payers are private and forty are public.

JG: How are you able to remain sustainable?

TA: It is the mission of the Beatitudes campus to serve the broader middle class. Our business plan is designed to manage the margin to serve the many. We have a variety of housing options that make our campus accessible.

JG: Do you charge residents a buy-in fee?

IH: Residents in independent living pay a buy-in fee. That price can range from two hundred and fifty to three hundred and fifty thousand dollars. They pay a monthly fee for services as well. We also have month to month rental units with no buy in requirement.

JG: When residents leave or pass away, do you reimburse any of the buy-in fee?

IH: Yes. Ninety percent is reimbursed to the resident or their family.

JG: What is the gender ratio of your residents?

TA: The residents are approximately one-third male and two-thirds female.

JG: Do the residents who are not living in the memory residences have memory issues?

TA: Their average age is eighty-seven. I estimate that sixty-five percent have trouble thinking. They live independently, but they have some cognitive challenges. We have services available to them as they age and their cognition declines.

KM: I know two nurses diagnosed with dementia a few years ago who were heartbroken when they had to stop working.

Luckily we have good diagnostic doctors in Phoenix. We are all or will all be touched by dementia in one way or another.

TA: We are designing a care model that will change many lives, including our own. The genetic make up of my children makes them more likely to develop dementia. My life's work will hopefully help them if need be. I want them to be treated with a sense of autonomy and to be allowed to fulfill their purpose.

JG: Do you think that it is a benefit for people to know if they have dementia?

TA: Yes. My family member was diagnosed early. It is a part of the human experience to be born to die. Believing that you can go on indefinitely is a fallacy based in denial. If a person is diagnosed, they can make a plan and lay out their priorities.

JG: Do you think that people do not want to be tested because of their fear of suffering?

TA: Maybe a person with dementia does not have to suffer. That is what Comfort Matters is about. If people are suffering, we are not doing our job. We have person centered interventions that alleviate suffering.

IH: Tena believes that we give Alzheimer's too much credit and too much power. There is no reason a person cannot be comfortable, even with dementia, through the end of their life.

TA: We know that dementia impacts your ability to think. That is unfortunate, and we all hope that we will eventually find a method to at least arrest its progression. Hopefully, one day we will eradicate dementia from the population entirely by treating everyone proactively in some way, such as by immunization. Our work and training is focused on how to make a comfortable life for someone who has already been diagnosed. We know that the brain is resilient, even with dementia. Parts of the brain, such as the emotional connection, are not as impacted as others. This is the reason that the way someone with dementia feels is far more important than the way they think. This is why we see such pronounced emotions in people living with dementia. The emotions lead the behaviors. The behaviors serve as communication when the words are difficult to find. If we can find ways to provide someone the ability to feel good, it does not matter that they cannot think.

IH: That is why music and art work so well. Music brings pleasure and often triggers memories. Music is a simple and powerful form of comfort.

TA: We know that the part of our brain that tells us when we are comfortable and when we are not is intact until our last breath. Our emotions are primarily intact. We can use that knowledge. If we know what makes someone comfortable and feel like they are in charge, they live well. We have done this and we can teach it. We have witnessed it being operationalized around the country.

KM: The reverse also holds true. Knowing what irritates people and eliminating it is a form of support. Irritants can include making a resident adhere to our schedule of waking and sleeping, making them eat food that we think they should eat, having a television on, using overhead pagers, requiring them to shower how and when we want them to shower, and using medical, emotional, and alarm restraints.

IH: That is why we do not have staff turnover in our dementia residences. They have positive and peaceful interactions with happy, comfortable residents.

JG: Please discuss staff turnover a bit more.

TA: We have employees who retire. We have people who are diagnosed with dementia. We have people who go back to school. That turnover is natural. Beatitudes Campus is a good place to work because our culture supports the employees.

IH: That is the empowerment piece of our culture. A few months ago we had guests from the Department of Health and Human Services. They were interested in learning about our Comfort Matters program at the Vermilion Cliffs memory residence. We had just finished telling the visitors that we empower our staff to engage and give comfort to the residents. When we arrived at the Vermilion Cliffs residence, an employee was stacking the laundry closet. Our resident, Terry Lee, was walking around with her earphones in and listening to music. As she passed the laundry employee, he turned around and took the time to dance with her and twirl her around. She had a big smile on her face. She was in heaven. We thanked the employee for taking the time to interact and connect with Terry. He responded, "I dance with her every day. I love it. That is why I come up here." That is part of the culture at Beatitudes. The empowerment of individuals. The laundry employee added joy and happiness to Terry's day and also to his own.

We have a resident who is not able to pronounce words. She is Hispanic. One day she appeared to be having a tough time and was sitting at a small table with her head down. A Hispanic maintenance man walked over, got down on his knees, looked her in the face, and started talking to her in Spanish. Her face lit up immediately. He chose to spend a little time to be with her and talk to her in her familiar language. Those interactions happen here regularly.

JG: What influenced the design of Comfort Matters?

TA: We began researching and designing the Comfort Matters program in 1997. The publications of Tom Kitwood were our early foundation and inspiration. Tom Kitwood promoted the concept of autonomy by identifying people as individuals, knowing them well, helping them to be comfortable, and recognizing that their behavior and their actions are their communication. Through our work, we learned that each member of the team must have the autonomy to help our residents to be comfortable, celebrate who they are, and feel a sense of well-being. If this responsibility is left to a couple of people or to part of our organization only, it does not work.

We began with weekly team meetings at Vermilion Cliffs, our advanced memory residence. We discussed each resident to determine their individual needs and preferences. We explored systems and structures that would support meeting those needs and preferences. Initially we learned that we were waking people at 4:30 or 5:00 in the morning for a 7:00 breakfast. Most of the residents are vulnerable and frail. This schedule was not focused on the needs of the residents. The schedule was built around our organizational goals. We examined and broke down some of those systems. We did this process as a team, including everyone from the housekeeper to the director. We compared our systems to the needs and preferences of the residents. We know that people with dementia generally do not sleep like everyone else; they must be afforded the opportunity to rest and relax when it makes the most sense to their bodies. If we honor their schedule then when they wake up they are in a much better mood, they are able to think more clearly, and they are able to do other activities more easily than they would if they were tired.

The team meetings were an important component to our research. We were able to design new systems and policies that supported each resident individually.

JG: What other challenges did you encounter in your culture change process?

KM: We had to challenge territorialism, not just the hierarchy and the chain of command. An example would be an employee thinking, "This is housekeeping. This is my realm. You cannot decide that we are going to readjust our schedule because people want to have access to food twenty four hours a day." We examined all of the systems that we had in place that supported territorialism and redesigned them. As we began implementing the new culture, we realized that it would take a total buy in from every employee and board member. Everyone had to recognize that the needs and preferences of the residents were directing our policies and procedures. The residents are guiding us by how they respond to issues. Who knows the residents best? The housekeeper who is in the room every day—not the management or the board.

Our job as managers is to support the entire staff in doing what they know to be best for the residents. Everyone understands that culture. There is no dictating downward. Management offers education and empowerment. I taught a senior staff member in class yesterday. I also had caregivers. The only top down sanction was that senior staff should encourage all of the employees in their department to bring any issues forward, to innovate, and to find special ways to connect to and create comfort for our residents.

We also have a fluid partnership with the families of our residents. We are continually exchanging information and collaborating with them to design a plan for their mom or dad. Situations change. Family members are an important part of our care team.

The business world does not naturally operate this way. This model demands one hundred percent employee participation and accountability. When we have discussions about changing a system and we hear, "It is going to interfere with my break" or "I will not be able to finish showering five residents," we are not happy. We want staff to understand that the choice was made for the comfort of the residents. Staff should adjust their schedules around the individual schedules of the residents. That is person directed culture.

JG: Why do you refer to yourselves as a campus?

TA: We were named Beatitudes Campus for a reason. This is a learning environment. We trial and we trial again. Sometimes we get it right. Sometimes we do not. The beauty of healing and medicine is that they incorporate art and science. Often providers are so focused on the science that they forget that art has to be considered in equal measure. We are elevating the art portion to the position it needs to be. There is an art to learning how to collectively develop ideas that keep the resident comfortable, autonomous, and in control.

JG: Was elevating the art portion a difficult process?

TA: We were able to develop beliefs and philosophies that did not necessarily support people. Why can we not develop policies, philosophies, and beliefs that do? We have experienced success in our training because we show people how to completely operationalize our philosophies and culture through an evidence based model.

KM: We tend the process. Person centered culture is fluid. We must keep modifying and adapting the process.

JG: Please describe some of your research.

TA: We are engaged in translational research. We have conducted two studies. One of them was in 2009. We completed another study more recently where we worked with three large nursing homes in New York. Comfort Matters palliative care implementation was at worst cost neutral; at best it created cost savings. There is no reason for an organization not to have an effective palliative care program. Our model uses very little or no antipsychotic medications and removes medications and exams that are no longer useful, such as prostate medications and mammograms.

IH: Additionally, we calculated that we saved thirty thousand dollars per patient per year by eliminating nutritional supplements that are no longer useful to the resident.

JG: Why do you think other memory care providers are not using the Comfort Matters model?

TA: The memory care industry is on the verge of changing the way care is delivered to everyone. This is new. When I presented at the Institute of Medicine and interacted with many people from around the country, I learned that there is a general philosophy about person directed living that most agree upon. The issue is how to operationalize the philosophy on a deeply cultural and sustainable level. We have been successful in translating the philosophy down to the finest details. It is embedded in every system and every employee. We have been training other organizations to do the same and have seen wonderful outcomes. Success does not come over night. We work for two years with our clients so that when we move on, person directed comfort is steeped in every aspect of their culture and operations.

JG: What other consistent outcomes have you witnessed with the implementation of Comfort Matters on the campus?

KM: Comfort Matters creates lower rates of incontinence and more toileting, minimal antipsychotic usage, no restraints, few alarms, no sundowning, an increased usage of pain medications (we use Tylenol), decreased hospitalizations, increased family and staff satisfaction, decreased staff turnover, and weight gain due to liberalized diets.

JG: Are people alarmed that you are not making the residents eat three balanced meals per day?

TA: The effectiveness of liberating the diet is not only our finding. The American Academy of Nutrition and Dietetics supports that position. They support eating whatever makes you happy whenever you wish.

JG: Is that a new position for the American Academy of Nutrition and Dietetics?

TA: No, they have been promoting liberalized diets since 2005. Their position was updated in 2012. That is what I show doctors when they prescribe an eighty-year-old Lipitor and put them on a cardiac diet.

JG: Has your research or experience shown which person would live the longest: the person who takes Lipitor and is on a cardiac diet or the person with no medications who eats whatever and whenever they want?

TA: Generally the person who eats what they want lives longer and in that time has a better quality of life.

JG: Are there safety issues when people want to eat at all hours?

TA: Most of the residents need ambulatory assistance. If a resident regularly likes to have a midnight snack, they will not be up walking around the kitchen alone. Staff understands that addressing this habit is part of their responsibility.

JG: Will the staff prepare a meal late at night?

KM: Yes. We have meals in the freezer that can be micro-waved. We see too much polypharmacy with our new residents. It takes us a while to start cutting back on the medications. Our medication average is four per person per day forever. That includes pain medication.

JG: Is that lower than the national average?

IH: It is much lower. The national average of medications taken by someone age sixty-five to seventy-nine is twenty. For those eighty and older that average is twenty-two.

TA: I had the opportunity to speak to the Institute of Medicine a couple of years ago. We told them about our medication rate. They were amazed. It seems like an obvious quality of life choice to us. When a person has a terminal condition and you give them many medications, they often cannot eat because they are full of medications. They also may not feel well because of the strength of the medications on their frail frame. It makes sense to start reducing the medications. We talk with families about Aricept and Namenda. The resident might have been taking medications for nine years and they might not be working much anymore, if at all. Now they are just creating expensive urine and uncomfortable stomachs. Liberalizing the diet often contributes to weight gain because the residents feel better and eat more.

JG: Are families hesitant to reduce the medications?

TA: Someone has to be brave and suggest medication reduction to the family and explain why. Families are usually ready and willing to lower medications.

KM: We want the right drug in the right dosage for the right person for the right reason. Some people need medication, but you must investigate all medication usage. There is an experimental nature to how we view everything. We are continually examining what works and what does not. When we take a medication away, we watch closely for any positive or negative effects. We see positive effects almost always. We carefully document and observe. The documentation helps us with the inspectors, as do our favorable health outcomes. Inspectors need to be certain that we are making choices that are safer and have better outcomes for our residents.

JG: Do you need more staff to make these medication changes?

KM: It is the opposite. Residents who are on fewer medications generally eat better, are happier, and are more stable. Their digestion works better too, which can make for better toileting. Another reason our residents do not need as much medication is because we let them live as they wish to the highest degree possible. We have one nurse for the thirty-eight people at Vermilion Cliffs. We need fewer staff because we use fewer medications and treatments, resulting in fewer calls to the doctors and fewer incident reports. We have four or five nursing assistants on days and evenings, depending on our situation. For example, if we have a new resident who is having trouble adjusting, we have more staff. As I mentioned earlier, ours is a fluid model based on the needs of the residents.

If you let people sleep as long as they like, they are far happier when we help them up out of bed. We need fewer staff when the residents are not angry that we woke them up and are forcing them out of bed. It is the same for eating, showering, and all other activities.

TA: We also use our entire staff to keep an eye on the residents. Our housekeepers are engaged. There is much more appeal to a housekeeping position when it is part of the caring environment. They are welcome to speak up for a resident. The rest of the staff appreciates the feedback and validates their concern and involvement. Our housekeepers are a valued part of the team and they know it.

IH: I love the story that Karen tells about one of our housekeepers.

KM: I was a nurse on the floor. One of the housekeepers asked, "Would you come and check on Mrs. M?" I asked, "Why?" She responded, "I do not want to tell you because you will think it is silly, but would you just check on her to make sure is she alright?" I conducted an assessment but nothing seemed amiss. I asked the housekeeper, "Please tell me what is different?" Her response was, "Mrs. M is not singing this morning." I answered, "Thank your for your feedback. We will watch her closely." The next day, Mrs. M spiked a temperature due to a urinary tract infection. The housekeeper, who listened to the resident singing each day, detected the early sign of discomfort. She knew the resident well. Importantly, the housekeeper knew that it was her place to voice her concern and that we would respond accordingly. We train many other managers around the United States. You would be surprised how few organizations include and understand the importance of feedback and connection between the housekeeper and all the other staff.

TA: They often remain an untapped resource.

IH: Our culture makes it easier to recruit people to work here. Our culture is also a marketing tool to attract residents. Because of our reputation, families want their family members to live here.

JG: Do you maintain the same staff at the same residences?

TA: Yes. There is a big push nationally for consistent staff assignments.

KM: The staff tells us what a big difference it makes. With consistent staff assignments, the families get to know the care partners and the other staff. This enables the families to be more involved and connected to the care. Organizations, including Beatitudes, who use consistent staff assignments have seen the number of family complaints drop or end all together.

TA: We had approximately one hundred data points in our research. We were not just determining whether it was cost effective for staffing. We measured hospitalization and emergency room visits.

We have had positive changes in all areas because an

117

empowered team works toward a common goal. There is a higher goal than just receiving a paycheck. Most people who work in healthcare are service minded. They do not stay in the industry if they are not. It is not about a job. We want to make a difference. We create the culture for the staff to experience making a difference and being part of a culture that is positive and life affirming.

KM: Our team also vets the products that we use. For example, we tried a different, thinner brief, but found that the cost savings were not what we had expected because we had to use more of them. Management can bring ideas, but the expertise and experience of the care team is more heavily weighted in decision making.

JG: How did you vet the briefs?

TA: I am proud to say every staff member participated in that process. We did have to tell a few family members that we looked a little extra padded because we were wearing briefs so we would understand the experience better. The families were quite impressed. I actually had a couple families offer to try them and report their experience, so I directed them to Walgreens where they could buy their own supply. Even though we were not all perfectly comfortable, the trial was well worth our time.

KM: We try many new ideas. We had residents in Adirondack chairs at one point. We had beanbag chairs another time. We used the Merry Walkers. We have learned to vet any product or system.

TA: When I began working at Beatitudes, we had many residents who were experiencing weight loss. Rather than accept weight loss as standard, we decided to carefully watch how people were eating. We learned that people were not eating or drinking their supplements. One day I collected a sample of every supplement the residents were taking and lined them all up. The staff tasted one or two supplements. That experience achieved full staff buy-in to stop feeding our elders unnecessary, bad tasting supplements that were likely making them feel full or nauseous or both.

KM: We challenge everything, but not all at once. We choose one subject at a time and then challenge the beliefs around the issue. We also examined bed rails. You may have noticed that we do not use bed rails. In one situation, we had a certified nursing assistant who was sure that one particular resident could move herself and insisted that we keep the bed rails. We stood watch outside the room for hours. She never moved, so we got rid of the bed rails.

JG: How did you determine your policy around restrictions other than bed rails?

TA: Our policy around restrictions is person directed.

KM: The policy is informed by the reaction of our residents.

IH: Our policies are based in knowing the person intimately. We also interview the family to learn what the resident was like before moving in, what kind of music they enjoy, and other personal preferences.

JG: Do you have locked doors in your memory care residences?

TA: We have secured doors, but what we use to secure the elevator is a red rope that implies that very important people live here. Buzzers, bells, and alarms are not consistent with comfort for people who have trouble thinking.

JG: Does the rope work?

KM: Yes. It has been very effective.

TA: The rope is also considerably cheaper than most other options that would create upset and distress.

KM: Our staff is highly engaged with the residents, so wandering off is not an issue for us.

TA: When we renovate, we will not have an elevator to contend with. The residents will always feel as though they are part of the community, and should not feel compelled to leave. For now, our care model must overcome bad design. There was no consideration of person directed dementia housing when the residence was built fifty years ago.

KM: In order to remove alarms and other restraints, all of the staff of the Beatitudes Campus must be included and updated. When we ran into problems with our elevators, we brought people in from the other departments. Anyone who gets off the elevator needs to know to wait until the elevator door closes and to not let a resident on. We want to ensure that employees do not unknowingly bring people downstairs. We examined all of the systems and detailed our policies in writing. The Comfort Matters culture is organization wide and involves each employee.

JG: How do you balance the less restrictive atmosphere of your dementia residences with the regulations?

TA: We understand that regulators come to their work just like we do—not knowing everything there is to know and having to learn. We never know whether or not they have had the opportunity to learn. Occasionally we have to convince the regulators. We seize the opportunity to educate regulators about what is important for the people we are serving because we are the experts. We can speak for the residents, and we need to speak for them. It would be unethical to fail to speak for them when we know what they need.

KM: The new guidelines for dementia are focused on person directed care and keeping people comfortable. An organization must put into place the policies and practices that support comfort and person directed care. All employees need dementia specific training. This creates the opportunity to dialogue and explain to inspectors and regulators why our care process is safer. It also enables our residents to experience the best quality of life possible. Our inspectors in Arizona are open to learning. They have spent a lot of time talking with staff. In the past, most regulatory concerns were brought to the director of nursing and the administrator. Today, regulators come in and speak to the housekeeper, the diet aide, and the nursing assistant. When an organization creates a team that has been empowered to do what they know needs to be done for the residents, the inspectors do not have to go to the higher level administration. The regulators see quality and comfort embedded in every fiber of the care. Our care team knows each person individually and can anticipate what gives them comfort and happiness. Our care culture is embedded in every person who interacts with the residents, which is almost everyone who works at Beatitudes Campus.

IH: Our culture is designed to empower the housekeepers, and all other members of the support system, to be able to make decisions along the way.

TA: When we began our work, we did not have as much of the confidence that we are showing you now. We have witnessed outcomes of our evidence based care model over many years. I have had a couple of advisory calls with the Centers for Medicare and Medicaid Services. They solicit our feedback to learn the best organizational practices for people in assisted living. Dementia does not know licensure. Our campus serves people at all levels of physical and cognitive ability. Some live in their own homes and others in skilled nursing, memory care, or assisted living. We are building strategies that support people where they are rather than strategies that add an extra layer of potential distress.

In the early stages of our culture transformation we ran into the "you cannot do that" response regularly. Change is generally met with resistance and fear. I suspect that is still the case in some organizations. We started to ask ourselves whether commonly held beliefs were fact or folklore. Beliefs such as, "you cannot have people eat whenever they want because the regulations will not let you" or "you have to have a nurse watch them as they eat even though the environment does not support good nutrition and a comfortable experience when they are with a group of people." Are these ideas fact or folklore? We learned that those and many others are folklore.

JG: How did you learn that these commonly held beliefs are folklore?

TA: We began this exploration in our early stages of culture change. We spoke regularly with the Health Department. I would ask, "Is this really a regulation? Could you direct me to the F-Tag?" F-Tags are guidelines for federal and state regulations. Sometimes the actual guideline can be different than what its interpretation has become over time. I researched many F-Tags.

KM: The organizations that we are training around the United States have done the same. They have built relationships with their regulators so that they can ask these kinds of questions and complete the groundwork ahead of time. The guides that are available are very well laid out. We learned to love the regulations.

We shared the guides with all of the departments so that we have the same information. When the guide for dementia specific care was designed, we shared it with our director of nursing.

She then met with her staff and they evaluated their processes. They made sure they were operationalizing person directed dementia care in every aspect of the residents' lives. We have learned to work within the framework of the regulations.

TA: We make our regulatory adherence transparent. We do not organize according to what we think might go wrong. We organize our system to meet the requirements of what is being asked in the regulations. That is the reason we commit to understanding both the letter and the spirit of the restrictions.

Occasionally the process is not perfectly smooth. We have said, "You are telling me this, but we do not agree and here is why. I will bring you the F-Tag and the scientific literature that supports this position." We have all of the research and F-Tags on hand for these conversations. We are prepared to have the research and other information that will allow the regulators to see things our way. Often, all we ever had to say was, "I have literature that supports our position. Would you like to see it?"

KM: Many surveyors have held other jobs previously. One is not required to attend school to be a surveyor. They understand the letter and are becoming better about the spirit of the regulations. Ten to fifteen years ago, surveyors were visiting and I was sitting and crocheting with a couple of ladies in the dementia living neighborhood. One resident was untangling as fast as I could crochet. We were sitting and talking about the arthritis in our fingers. Another staff member was reading the paper to someone. Another was sitting in the common area and another was styling someone's hair. There were approximately five different activities happening. The surveyor asked, "Where is your activity?"

IH: They were looking for group activity.

TA: They said, "That is not what we are expecting to see."

We explained that everyone was involved in an activity and it was fine. Person directed activities are those that the resident feels like doing, not some class type structured activity that we impose upon them.

IH: We recently met our resident Terry Lee and Mr. Shubundi from our dementia living residence out on the putting green. That is an activity. Regulators had to be told that activities can be broken up into small groups. Terry Lee and Mr. Shubundi walked across the campus to the putting green and interacted with other residents and with all of us in the process. Then they practiced their golf. I do not know that you would see that situation in many other life course living communities.

TA: Terry Lee was formerly an executive for Marriott and likes to inspect for problems. She will comment, "That needs to be painted. Why is that not being taken care of? You know that plant needs watering." This behavior is ingrained in her nature.

KM: When we bring guests to the Vermilion Cliffs, she wants to make sure we are taking care of them to her standards.

TA: She will let us know if she thinks that we have not done what we should. We have a culture where she is free to be her supervisor self.

KM: That is just it. Even those living with dementia are individual people. Most of our residents come in with sixty-five or more years of life behind them. We honor that life and the person they are because of their life experience. We must have a culture that allows people to be themselves. That is the heart of person directed living.

JG: Do you have any intergenerational activities?

TA: We partner with several of the schools in the area. One is Washington High School, which is just down the street. They bring the students here for service projects. We designate a student of the month. We also honor the Washington High School students with a big banquet at the end of the year where we award scholarships.

JG: Are the residents involved in those events?

TA: Our residents decide who wins. They also donate the scholarship funds. We have many retired teachers who live here. Our campus is based in purposeful living. On our campus, there are over ninety-seven clubs and meetings that were started by residents and are resident run.

IH: Every Wednesday night we have a Hootenanny on campus. Igor Glenn organizes the Hootenanny. He is a musician who was formerly with the New Christy Minstrels. The New Christy Minstrels were a group of twelve to fifteen people that produced many popular songs. He still travels all over the world. Every Wednesday, people come from all over the community with their instruments to participate in the Hootenanny.

TA: They are professional musicians.

IH: Some of them live on the Beatitudes Campus and others are from outside the campus. Some of them decided to live here because of the Hootenanny.

TA: We also have an active resident run group, Seniors for a Sustainable Future, who have lobbied in Washington, DC. We have residents who have spent their lives making contributions to the broader community, which is why many of our groups are civic minded.

JG: Being a faith-based organization, are the Beatitudes residents diverse in lifestyle and religion?

TA: Did you see our sign our front that says, "Open to business for everyone"? We were the first organization in Arizona that was publicly open and affirming to people of all lifestyles.

We are very proud of that. We believe that everyone has a place at the table. We had a number of residents who wanted to more fully connect with the lesbian, gay, bisexual, and transgender community. They contacted the people who operate PFLAG, which is a group that supports the lesbian, gay, bisexual, and transgender community and their friends and families. Today, they meet on campus weekly. We recently screened the movie *Gen Silent* on the campus. Our lesbian, gay, bisexual, and transgender support group has approximately one hundred fifty members.

IH: We hold many activities for the community, including AARP, Alzheimer's groups, and other support groups. The Beatitudes residents are welcome to attend all the community activities.

JG: Please describe your home based services.

KM: We provide a variety of home health services through our Beatitudes at Home and Beatitudes Home Health programs. Our caregivers offer support to our campus residents and to those in their homes in the local community.

TA: We are a life plan community without walls.

JG: How have you eliminated sundowning in your dementia residences?

TA: People who have trouble thinking have specific needs. They need to be able to sleep when they are tired. They need to eat what they want and when they want. They need to receive assistance with the activities of daily living in a way that is meaningful and appropriate to them—not convenient for us but for them. They need to be engaged in ways that are meaningful and that celebrate who they are as people. Their environment should exist to support them. Someone who cannot think well generally cannot tolerate a lot of noise and commotion. They cannot make sense of it. They think, "I am uncomfortable and afraid and do not know what to do." Loud, unpredictable, institutional type culture is noxious to those with thinking problems. If we help people sleep when they are tired and wake when they are refreshed, they are often their best self. We have to anticipate their needs and know each individual well enough that we know when they are hungry or thirsty. If their stomach is aching because they are hungry, they are not going to be able to tell us. If we are mindful in managing these aspects, the likelihood that someone will sundown is substantially reduced.

Reducing sundowning is also achieved with medication management or reduction. For example, nine hours after someone receives an antipsychotic, anxiolytic, or Ativan, that person experiences what is referred to as a hangover effect. They feel like they had too much to drink. When practitioners give a medication to someone that makes them feel bad nine hours later, this sets up the conditions that create the anxiety and unhappiness that lead to sundowning. When a person has difficulty thinking and feels sick or hungover most of time, they are prone to sundowning.

IH: Tena just explained the engagement part of the Comfort Matters culture. If an older resident with dementia begins fixating on picking their children up from school, we find ways to calm them that do not involve drugging them. Another phrase I enjoy hearing Tena say often is, "We like to give their brain a better offer."

TA: We have been engaged in many behavioral consultations in Phoenix and all over the country. We have found that boredom is almost always a factor in sundowning. Many people still do not understand that the start button is broken for those with dementia.

JG: Do they need to be engaged?

127

TA: They do not want to just be sitting there, but they are unable to move to the next step. Their brain will not allow them. Someone has to be the kick starter. When we make their brain a better offer, we are offering them something of value; something other than frustration and boredom. They cannot verbalize it but they are thinking, "Thank you. I was just waiting for you to help me out." If we can anticipate the need for a start, we can prevent a resident from becoming frustrated. Frustration is how they communicate that they need a kick start if we have missed the cues. At such times, we give them a start, not a pill. This is a non-pharmacological measure that is much more effective most of the time.

IH: A kick start will differ from person to person. Someone might want a chocolate bar or an ice cream sandwich. Someone might want to get up and walk around. Someone else might want to knit and feel the texture of the yarn in her fingers.

TA: Another resident may just want to spend time with you because they see you as family or as a friend.

JG: Is preventing the agitation in essence what enables you to stop using the antipsychotic medications?

KM: Everyone, including us, has the potential for sundowning. People living with dementia do not have the same tolerance for boredom and agitation. We are mindful of tolerance.

TA: A person with memory issues cannot reason. They are not able to say to themselves, "Oh it is alright. I just need to sit here a few minutes and they will bring me something to eat. Then this pain in my belly will go away. I can wait. It is not a big deal. Let me distract myself by looking at this magazine."

JG: Someone living with dementia does not have tolerance for delayed gratification?

TA: Right. When they have needs, they need them met

immediately. When the care team deeply knows the residents, they do not wait until a resident is agitated. The care team identifies the need and prevents the delaying of gratification.

JG: What are your thoughts on preventing falls?

KM: Meeting the needs of a person is the most important and effective way to prevent falls.

TA: Exactly. Why do you pop up out of a chair? You are hungry or bored or need to use the toilet. When the care team notices that someone is "rejecting care," there are two options. The provider can contact the doctor and be given a prescription to calm the resident or understand the reason for the agitation and address the need. Here, if a resident is "resisting care," we determine the cause. We might suspect that their arthritis is more painful today because it is humid. We would change the dosage of their Tylenol and observe. We do not need to call the doctor to make the resident comfortable.

KM: Calling the doctor is a last resort.

TA: Yes. Absolutely.

JG: How do you walk the line between dignity and risk?

TA: You saw two of our later stage memory residents practicing their golf on your way in. Would you have known they have memory challenges if we had not told you?

JG: No. You are not concerned that they might fall over the ball or trip during the walk over to the putting green?

KM: They have support from the activities person who accompanied them.

TA: Think about it—humans fall. It is the threat of litigious activity that blocks organizations from enabling a person to experience freedom and quality of life. We consult with the decision makers. We tell the family that an activity is vital to their parent's experience in life, because this is what their parents have always done. When the family agrees, we share the responsibility for that risk.

JG: Do you also find that you are educating the families?

TA: Most people do not understand the progression of dementia. We continue to educate and inform the families with an ongoing dialogue. Karen mentioned partnering with the families. We see the families as our partners. That is essential. If we do not partner with the families then they will never understand the best choices for their parents. Often, this is their first experience with dementia. We have experience with thousands of people living with dementia. We are there to guide them throughout the time their parent is living with us.

KM: This is informed consent.

TA: Yes, at its highest calling.

JG: Which of your staff are trained in Comfort Matters?

KM: Every employee is trained in the Comfort Matters culture. We host an orientation for all of our new employees about Comfort Matters, what is expected of the employee on campus, and how employees should approach the residents. After orientation, employees attend either a two hour or eight hour monthly training. All employees working specifically in the memory neighborhood, the department managers, and the supervisors attend the monthly eight-hour training. We continually educate and invest in our human capital.

JG: Even the grounds staff is trained in Comfort Matters?

KM: Absolutely. Each of our four hundred and twenty-five employees are engaged in continual training. I am the Comfort Matters nurse educator for the campus. We are conducting Comfort Matters training around the country, but we have maintained a strong dedication to our employees on this campus. Tena and I teach the eight-hour training.

JG: Please describe the Comfort Matters training program that you are providing throughout the United States.

IH: When we began to teach the Comfort Matters model, Tena taught other organizations on a train the trainer model.

TA: It was not as easy for people to make the necessary changes with education alone, then being sent off on their own. There was no one to guide them through the operational steps.

IH: We give a two hundred and fifty page education manual to every organization that is involved with our Comfort Matters training. You might say, "This is proprietary material. Why would you share it freely?" But the knowledge alone is not enough. To operationalize the knowledge and model, an organization needs hands on support over a long period of time. The training is always evolving.

Presently, we have fourteen client organizations that are participating in our Comfort Matters training. We have coaching calls with them every week or every other week, depending on how long they have been in training.

Our newest client is the Actors Home in New Jersey.

JG: Are you teaching them how to implement your dementia living model?

IH: Yes. They are a Comfort Matters provider now.

JG: Are you training the housekeepers too?

TA: Yes. We have manuals specific to each position, including housekeepers.

IH: When we begin a new consultation, we spend a week with them at their organization.

TA: We spend a considerable amount of time preparing before that first week. We talk with the management to determine how we can support them through the process, because change is difficult. Karen and I or Karen and Linda Travis and I will learn the priorities of the management and draft the agenda for week one. We customize the plan according to the individual needs of the organization. Generally, we spend the first day getting to know the care team and make observations in their neighborhood. We teach to the strengths of each team member and identify opportunities for change to make comfort more available to the residents. On the first day, we will look for signs that a resident may be in pain. Pain is under-recognized and undertreated for those living with dementia.

JG: Is that because they cannot verbalize the fact that they are in pain?

TA: Yes.

JG: How does one recognize that someone living with dementia is in pain?

TA: There are reliable tools available. They just need to be used as part of the model of care. Positioning is another issue, as is boredom. We examine all the factors that could make someone uncomfortable and determine how that discomfort is communicated, or better yet, prevented. We begin to build relationships with the staff as the training progresses. Eventually, the care team will start to find their way with our education, support, and guidance. We do not go in as dictators. We will be working with them for two years. We offer two separate eight-hour education sessions during the next two days. We guide the care partners in directions. We may ask, "Did anyone notice that Mr. J was in pain?"

KM: We will solicit their observations.

IH: Tena and Karen establish the baseline or benchmark the first week and construct a plan from that point.

TA: Change happens in many ways. It is important for us to get a good baseline on the first day. Then we conduct two one-day eight-hour education sessions. Our education is multi-modal in that there is didactic education, video, discussion, case studies, and exercises.

This model is evidence based. The workforce that we are training across the country is made up of people from many different cultural backgrounds. The multi-modal approach allows for the greatest understanding. We at Beatitudes hail from twenty-seven different countries, and speak over ninety percent of the languages of the world.

We spend the first two days meeting the staff where they are. We continue to build our relationships with them so they understand that we are not adversarial. We present them with information that they likely never knew. We may also be verifying and vetting things that they already knew to be good care but that the system did not support.

KM: Many of the staff we train is happy to have us. We are telling our story. They are telling their story. Even in the education we are making those bonds.

TA: On the first evening, we may bring an example from the day so the staff can examine it. We really use their strengths and their opportunities in framing the education. We think that process is unique. We believe that is the best opportunity for learners that we can give them. At the end of the day on Thursday, after we have done the education, we have a learning circle. Accountability and involvement are vital to success. We go around the circle and ask everyone what they have learned. That is a moment of realization for them. We ask what each person learned that will influence them to revise one process the next day. We teach, the participants have realizations, and they make the changes.

KM: They tell their peers, bosses, and everyone else in the room that they are planning to make specific changes.

TA: There is beautiful symmetry to it. We provide teaching and a safe enough environment for people to realize that they may not have been providing the best care, and help them pave a path to do so. We have some people who break down and say, "I had it all wrong and now I understand." The staff describes the process as rewarding. People working with the elderly generally want to create the best possible lives for them. We help them attain that wish.

KM: At one of our organizations, we had a maintenance man stop to thank us. He was happy to become part of the team.

TA: On Thursday, after we have done the education and sharing circle, we send the staff off to apply all of their learning and realizations.

KM: We work together with them in the application.

TA: The staff is often excited to try new methods. Sometimes they will tell us, "That person is suffering so much. I cannot believe I had not noticed the signs before. Now I know I can fix it. I have the tools. I know they hurt. I know that they are rejecting care because they have arthritic pain." Those moments are exciting for us all. We work as a team to create comfort. It is rewarding for the staff to have calm, comfortable residents.

KM: We work with many departments, including the activity department and the social department, to help them become part of the transformation.

JG: Do you see recurring themes from organization to organization?

KM: We see similar themes in every group. We expect to see issues regarding the treatment of pain. We also usually have team dynamics to address.

TA: Our model is being continually validated when we witness the transformations.

JG: Themes you have mentioned are pain, sundowning, and team dynamics. Are there other themes that you commonly address in your training?

KM: Positioning.

JG: Does positioning mean how you sit someone?

KM: Positioning refers to how people are sitting, what they are sitting in, how long they are sitting, and how liberalized their routines are.

The Comfort Matters concept is based in how the team orchestrates what to do and when to do it. The staff is often stuck in a routine designed to accomplish their responsibilities. We pry that process open with them and examine how much of the plan is based around the needs of the residents. Sometimes the processes and schedules are too rigid. One example is requiring everyone to be in the dining room from noon until one. Residents have to move whether they are done or not because the dining people have to start cleaning up. This creates an elevated stress level with residents reacting to caregivers and housekeepers rushing the process of eating, which should be pleasurable and relaxing.

TA: Or the overhead pager is going off.

KM: Noise is often another theme. If they have overhead pagers or other alarms, it is an issue that we will deal with. From the beginning of working with a new client, we immediately start seeing patterns. Some organizations have worked on diets and supplements before we arrive. Some organizations use far too many antipsychotics and anxiolytics. The usage varies from state to state.

TA: We check the statistics before we go so we have a sense of what we will be facing. We look at their Centers for Medicare and Medicaid Services filings also. On the last day of the first intensive week, we sit down with members of the team and create a strategic plan for moving forward. We ask them where they believe they have opportunities to enhance comfort. We help them with the list. We also help to prioritize the list. Next, we help them to establish structures for communication. Good communication is vital.

JG: Are you referring to communication to the resident from the care partner?

TA: All communication is important, including communication with us because we have coaching calls. In the early process, we have a weekly thirty-minute coaching call.

IH: Before Tena and Karen leave on Friday, the weekly coaching calls are scheduled.

JG: In this two-year process, what happens after the first week other than the coaching calls?

TA: This is where we differ from some of the other more prescriptive programs. The culture of each organization is unique to them, including who they serve and where they are located. We help them recognize what direction they should move and we help them get there. Our process is not prescriptive in any way. We do not have a rigid timeline.

JG: What do you discuss in the weekly call?

TA: We gently and kindly guide our clients. Earlier this week I was on a call with a fairly new organization. They were evaluating dining for comfort. I began by asking them about the process. We learned that management and housekeeping had embraced the model but that the nursing and food service teams had not. I asked why they were not adopting the new model. They responded, "Some of them are reluctant to change." Culture change will not happen in a divided team. Our contract is for two years, so we have time to work this early issue out.

KM: Sustainability is at the forefront of our minds when we work with the clients who are implementing Comfort Matters. If they fail in sustaining the Comfort Matters model, we have failed. From the first day of our training, we begin impressing the need for continuing education for every member of the care team. Organizations must make continuing education a part of their policy. We give them all the materials they need. We expect that each member on their team will complete the core competencies. Some organizations begin with the memory neighborhood and then bring it outward in layers to the other staff. However, if they have a housekeeper and a relief housekeeper or anyone else who is in the memory neighborhood, they too must have their competencies completed. They can provide the continuing education in their weekly team meeting or in other creative ways. One group hosts Comfort Fairs that they have periodically scheduled in addition to their education.

We adapt our teaching to the competencies of the care team and the individual needs and issues of the organization. All of the staff must be engaged. When we return, we will be able to see it. They also must be able to explain the process of implementation to us. We leave them with the educational materials and nurture their transition on the coach calls. We have one group that has been working with Comfort Matters for approximately four months. They are doing very well with their transition. I told them that in about another three weeks, our calls would become bimonthly rather than weekly. They were not happy because they have become reliant on our weekly calls as an accountability of sorts.

JG: Are the coaching calls mostly you advising?

KM: We say very little during the coaching calls. We listen as they work through a process.

TA: We facilitate the process, which is about them, not about us. Most people want to do a good job and are committed to working out the kinks. Comfort Matters does two things: it helps change staff practice through competency building— we build competency toward dementia appropriate care—and it also helps organizations change their systems of operation. Both aspects are necessary.

JG: Could you give an example of system change?

TA: When we address dining systems, an organization might be serving fifty people in their dementia neighborhood. The common thought is that you are feeding fifty people. That is wrong. You are feeding one person, and you may have to do that fifty different ways. How do you create flexibility in your systems so that fifty people can all eat differently? They eat different foods, at different times, in different locations, and in different amounts.

KM: The kitchen here at Beatitudes expects a variety of food orders at a variety of times. The food supervisor is part of the training, so it begins to make sense to them why the system is being changed. The supervisor must create a system that supports the staff in supporting the resident.

JG: What communication, other than the weekly or bimonthly calls, do you have with your clients?

IH: Our clients provide us with monthly data. They maintain a chart that shows the use of a tool called PAINAD, which is measured against rejection of care. We want to see the use of PAINAD increase—because they are monitoring people in pain—and the rejection of care decrease. All of that is measured.

JG: What pain medications do you usually use?

IH: Tylenol.

JG: How do you convince the management of organizations that they will realize a return on investment for the cost and time of the Comfort Matters implementation?

IH: We do not ever guarantee results. Comfort Matters implementation has been cost neutral for the organizations we have trained. Our consultant calculated that Comfort Matters implementation resulted in a thousand dollar increase in value per resident per month. We charge our training clients sixty dollars per resident per month for two years.

JG: After you have completed the first week of training and the weekly and bimonthly calls, how do you continue to evaluate and train the organizations that you work with?

IH: Six months into the training, one of our educators returns to the campus to evaluate and fine tune policies and procedures based on the individual needs of the organization. After approximately a year, we return to conduct an accreditation survey. This is an essential aspect of the training program. Two educators return to measure the ability of the organization to demonstrate that they have embedded Comfort Matters into their practices. The educators ask questions and observe. Once the provider is accredited, we give them a plaque stating that they are a Comfort Matters provider. Accreditation lasts for one year. They also get camera ready art that they can put on their website stating that they are an accredited Comfort Matters provider. We also provide a press release that they can customize to their needs. Six months after accreditation, we return to determine their needs. We continue coaching calls every other week until we reach the two-year mark. We have been consulting in Comfort Matters for a year and a half. We have two organizations that have completed their accreditation. They have both asked for pricing to continue with us beyond two years. They are already seeing the value of the program.

TA: We have clients who are dedicated to person directed care but do not look good in their Centers for Medicaid and Medicare records. They want to fix the problems but honestly do not know how to do so. Last week I was at an organization and one of the certified nursing assistants ran up to me and said, "I just want to talk to you. I just want to thank you." And I said, "What are you thanking me for?" She replied, "Because you gave me tools. I am so happy. We can care for the residents in the way we have always wanted and hoped. It has made all the difference."

JG: Do they ever come up with innovative methods of implementation that you had not thought of?

TA: They do. That is one of the amazing outcomes. When that happens, we connect one organization to another.

KM: We might link a dietician in one organization who has wonderful ideas with another dietitian across the country. They can exchange best practices.

TA: One organization that just started in June made a bulletin board to post their successes. In their weekly team meetings they highlight all of the successes of the week. This reinforces that change is possible. I often receive permission to share their stories with other organizations.

KM: Some organizations have invited us to present with them. They want to share their story and to gain the recognition of their peers for their accreditation and culture change success. It is meaningful to have a group of organizations that are touting their success at sustaining Comfort Matters. This shows that it is possible.

TA: We love when people from the organizations we are training stand up and tell their stories. They become experts themselves over time. We recently returned from the Pioneer Network where Karen, our colleagues from New York, and I did a three-and-a-half-hour seminar. Then Comfort Champions came up and talked about their specific experiences. Brought the house down.

KM: When people learn that more organizations are successfully practicing Comfort Matters and experiencing positive outcomes, they might think it is possible for them. It is easy for an organization to think it is not possible because they have more challenging residents or they cannot afford the implementation. We all struggle to enable the best possible lives for our residents, and we all have the potential to shift to person directed care.

JG: Do your clients measure any outcomes of the implementation?

TA: We measure emergency department visits and hospitalizations. We have been implementing and researching Comfort Matters here for eighteen years, but we have been teaching others for twelve. Comfort Matters is a culmination of what we have learned from all of our experiences. From the beginning we decided to measure outcomes of cost and the quality of life of each person. Those of us who have worked in care service understand that if we are not focusing on the person when evaluating outcomes, we have missed the point. For example, what is the quality of life of a person who is drugged and dazed and sitting in a wheelchair alone all day? That person would never fall or become agitated, but they would have no quality of life or comfort in living. Data measure is important in the evaluation and affirmation of the program. Facts are useful with our board and our grantors.

JG: Have the organizations that you are training witnessed decreased staff turnover?

KM: Yes. We have experienced lower turnover rates of the line staff.

TA: We are not conducting traditional translational research with all of the organizations we train because that would add another layer of staff. We have conducted research with three organizations in the New York City area: the New Jewish Home, the Isabel Geriatric Center, and Cobble Hill Life Care. From this research, we collaborated with CaringKind to produce the Palliative Care for People with Dementia Guidelines.

JG: What do you charge for the two-year Comfort Matters consultation?

IH: We charge ten thousand dollars to start that first week. Then we charge sixty dollars per resident bed at a minimum of twenty-five beds. Once they become accredited, our fee drops to fifty dollars per resident bed and we continue on with coaching calls and all the other support. We do not charge them for extra calls or additional support requests. After two years, organizations have the opportunity to sign a renewal contract.

JG: Do you stay in a hotel for the first week site visit?

IH: We may stay in a hotel or on their campus with the residents.

TA: Which is always so much fun.

IH: We would rather stay with the residents if we can.

JG: Is the Comfort Matters model more expensive to maintain than the older and more industrialized models?

IH: That is important. The organizations that we have trained have realized better health outcomes and cost savings. They have also found that the savings have made the implementation cost neutral. With no margin, there is no mission.

TA: I would like to show you a short video. Less than two hundred people have seen this. This is one of our residents, Joanne.

> [Audio from video]
> JOANNE (J): . . . and some people have lost hope. Can I help with the hope bit?
> CAREGIVER (C): What?
> J: Can I help with the hope bit?
> C: You give hope every time you smile, Joanne.
> [End video]

Joanne helps with hope all the time. That is what this work is. It is hopeful work. It is being able to do something that serves people in a more profound way. It is hopeful for us. It is hopeful for them. It is hopeful for their families.

JG: Thank you for sharing the video and thank you for this interesting discussion.

KM: Thank you.

IH: Thank you for coming to Phoenix.

TA: Thank you for your interest in Beatitudes Campus and Comfort Matters.

— END OF INTERVIEW —

St. John's Case Study

An interview with **Rebecca Priest**

Background

St. John's has four senior living campuses in Rochester, New York, offering a variety of housing options including independent and assisted living, rehabilitation, and long-term care. Their four campuses include Brickstone by St. John's, St. John's Meadows, St. John's Home, and two Green House homes.

Brickstone by St. John's independent living community is located within a larger neighborhood in an urban setting and is home to more than one hundred residents. The Brickstone campus is laced with paths and trails for walking and biking. Brickstone has the look and feel of a village. Central to the community is the Village Square, which has dining, retail, meeting, and event spaces. Residents have the option to live in a bungalow, an apartment, or a town house-style home.

St. John's Meadows is another independent living campus, situated on a thirty-five acre property. Residents can choose to live in a cottage or apartment with meals and other supportive services available as needed. This campus is close to shops, restaurants, and healthcare providers, enabling the one hundred and thirty-nine residents to stay engaged in the neighborhood.

The St. John's Home campus is home to four hundred and fifty-five residents. It is the first nursing home in Rochester to become Eden

Alternative certified, which means that management and staff are committed to a model of care called person directed long-term living. This model of care encourages connected relationships between care partners and elders to improve the quality of life for both. St. John's Home is transforming an older, clinical building into twenty-two small homes, one floor at a time. The remodeled floors contain two residences each that resemble penthouse apartments with a kitchen and large living room.

Finally, St. John's boasts two Green House homes located within the Penfield suburban neighborhood. Each is home to around ten residents. It is impossible to distinguish these skilled nursing homes from the other houses in the community.

In this interview, Rebecca Priest details the path to operationalizing the Eden Alternative philosophies and implementing the Eden Alternative culture.

About Rebecca Priest

Rebecca Priest serves as the Administrator of Skilled Nursing at St. John's Home. She has held this role since 2013. She previously worked in social work roles at Heritage Christian Services and ROHM Services. Ms. Priest studied at the State University of New York at Buffalo toward becoming a Licensed Master of Social Work and has a Nursing Home Administrator's License.

INTERVIEW

Jean Galiana (JG): Please tell me what spurred your CEO, Charlie Runyon, to embrace the Eden Alternative principles and model of long-term care.

Rebecca Priest (RP): Charlie grew up in the tiny town of Sherburne, New York. It is the same town that Bill Thomas is from. Charlie worked at a local nursing home, Chase Memorial, which is where Bill and Jude Thomas eventually started the Eden Alternative. He spent most of his time running activities and helping people move from one place to another. He loved connecting with elders. That is where Charlie's passion for this industry began.

Charlie came to St. John's with the culture of connection in his DNA. When he first arrived, we were not being trained in the Eden Alternative. About twelve years ago, one of our doctors met with Charlie and said, "I am burned out. I cannot do this anymore. We have to make changes. This is what I want to do. I want to connect with Eden Alternative. I want to do something better than what I am doing here now as a physician." Charlie was easily convinced. We trained our entire leadership staff. We worked with our board and began the Eden Alternative path to mastery. We worked closely with the Eden Alternative to begin our culture change. I have worked with Charlie for fourteen years. He is a true leader. Charlie does not micromanage. He hires people who have a passion and fire to provide great care and he lets them innovate. I would not have the ability to convert an existing legacy structure and organizational culture to the Eden Alternative and small home model without Charlie Runyon at the helm.

Charlie runs our entire organization. He oversees me and I oversee skilled nursing. He also oversees the Meadows and Brickstone and he supports our board. Charlie is the chief executive officer and I am the Administrator of Skilled Nursing for St. John's Home.

JG: Please describe your process of converting to the Eden Alternative philosophies and the small home or Green House environment.

RP: We have a small home setting in both of our long-term care campuses. We are converting our urban campus from an older style environment to a small house setting based on the Eden Alternative philosophies. We also have Penfield, our suburban campus, which has two certified Green House homes. The homes are certified much like a brand name. Our two Green House residences have access to the outdoors. They also have private rooms and private showers. Residents share the space and eat together at the large dining room. Those aspects of the physical environment are trademarks of a Green House home.

It is much more difficult to achieve the small home setting on our urban campus because of the costs of retrofitting an existing institutional structure. Because of these limitations, we cannot meet the brand guidelines for a certified Green House home so, instead, we create a small home. No more than twenty elders reside in each small home. We have a built environment filled with cues to remind the residents that they are in their house. It is their space. It is not a medical space that belongs to a nursing team or a medical team. It is not an institutional space that residents have to stay in but which belongs to someone else. It is their space. The pace of the day is set by the elders who live in the house. The house elders determine the activities and priorities. We strive to remind residents that they are in their own home. Residents bring their own furniture for their individual rooms. They are also encouraged to bring some favorite items to decorate the common spaces, like a piece of art, a vase, or photographs. The residents make the decisions on design changes.

JG: How do you involve residents in the design decisions?

RP: We work with an interior designer who brings in photographs of possible designs. She asks the residents for their input and does her best to merge everyone's preferences. We also include the design preferences of family members. This is another way to ensure that residents know it is their home. When residents know they are living in their own home, they feel comfortable hanging a picture that is meaningful to them.

Their family may say, "It would really help mom reminisce if you put out the book from our trip to Ireland." The home reflects the residents.

We also use other non-institutional design choices. For example, our call lights resemble wall sconces. We do not have an overhead light that dings and flashes red. Residents have medicine cabinets just like you or I have in our bathrooms. You could call it elder friendly or dementia friendly, but we just call it common sense. Glaring red lights and beeping can be disturbing to someone with dementia, but they are also disturbing to everyone else.

Residents use hand towels instead of paper towels. We did some research and found that people like to keep hand towels in nice baskets to be used individually, like at the spa. We make sure that they are washed regularly. Residents and families are able to do their own laundry in the house if they wish. Having the ability to do laundry has been a big advantage for residents. They can wash personal items the way they want them washed. We forget how many simple things people lose when they move into a nursing home. I am very particular about how I do my laundry. Most of us are. Most of us learned how to do it from our mother. One of the things we ask our elders when they move in is how they like to do their laundry. Some people like to hang everything to dry and some people like to have it go through the dryers. Some people like to iron their laundry. We regularly ask ourselves, "Would I put this in my own home?" when considering design options. There is a way to make a warm, welcoming, and inclusive environment while meeting the challenges of regulations.

The families of our residents know that they do not need permission but rather are encouraged to do activities that they would like to with their loved ones at home. Perhaps they want to make dinner with their mom or cookies with their dad. This model allows the family to be involved in caring and interacting with their loved one like they would at home.

We have double beds like you and I would have at home. They are residential. They are not hospital beds. They are one height and the head and feet come up like an adjustable bed. What we have seen is a great reduction in falls from bed and much healthier sleeping patterns. It is hard for me to know whether the outcomes are due to the actual bed structure or the warm homelike environment the beds foster.

Most of our care partners do not wear scrubs or any other uniforms. We encourage care partners to wear their regular clothing.

JG: During our site visit, I was trying to decide who was working and who was not.

RP: That is beautiful. That is the goal. Care partners look like family. Some people are really afraid of breaking down that barrier. We are struggling with that on our urban campus. Some staff still wear scrubs because they want to. They think they will be dishonored and devalued otherwise. Uniforms are not necessary here because residents and families know who the care partners are. Care partners have deep and lasting relationships with the families and the residents.

Shifting from uniforms to regular attire is one of the stepping stones for culture change. Culture change requires the investment of time to achieve employee understanding. Our culture is based on the Eden Alternative philosophies. When staff members understand the philosophies, the changes make more sense. We will revisit uniforms again in six months. We will talk with elders about this dress issue.

No care partners wear scrubs in Penfield. Penfield was a newly built home that was steeped in the Eden Alternative philosophies and the Green House structure from the start. The care partners were not working in a legacy organization and then asked to change their way. They volunteered to move into this environment and wanted to change. Some of the staff are happy to have the opportunity to express themselves with casual, professional attire.

JG: Are those without scrubs or uniforms formally trained health professionals?

RP: Yes. They are all nurses and certified nurse assistants. The research regarding uniforms suggests that when elders see people in scrubs, they actually act sicker. They expect to have more done for them. When you are working with someone who is dressed in a nice shirt and slacks, people do as much for themselves as possible and do not feel as sick. We have observed that elders will try to do a lot more for themselves, like trying to move out into the garden or going to the kitchen for a snack. We see a lot less of that helplessness than they do in the older style institutions. The no uniforms policy is especially helpful for people living with dementia because they might forget that they are in a nursing home. They are just living among other people.

JG: What have you noticed about the rates of antipsychotic use by your residents since you converted to the Eden Alternative philosophies and the Green House environment?

RP: This is a tricky number because we have to factor in the individual elder and what he or she is already taking. You cannot move someone in and say, "We do not use antipsychotics here," and expect them to stop on the spot. It does not work that way. Every person we have moved into Penfield was on a typical antipsychotic. We took in people who needed a different option than traditional long-term care. These houses typically are not for people who are the best behaved and the most wealthy with the most supportive families.

We had one hundred percent antipsychotic use for the first

three months. Only two years ago, we had a twenty-three percent rate of antipsychotic use. That was still too high. We are now at fifteen percent across all of our residences. This is a great reduction in the last two years. Five percent of the residents of our Green Houses use antipsychotic medications.

I would love to see our rate go to zero. But I also know the type of elder who moves into our homes and I understand the struggles that they have in traditional homes. Usage varies because people are regularly moving in. That means one person living in the Green House takes antipsychotics. Often they are with us because of mental health issues. We still count those residents in our antipsychotic outcome measurement.

We have not put anyone on antipsychotics. Because of our culture, we are able to take most residents off of them. We create interventions to "bad behaviors," which we see as reactions to unmet needs. We try to identify the needs and find better alternatives to address them.

JG: How did you build small homes in an existing, old fashioned structure?

RP: Our urban home is a typical 1970s institution. The floors that are unmodified are in the shape of the letter H with the elevator in the center and two long, narrow, institutional hallways on either side. The rooms of the residents are off the hallways, similar to a clinical or hospital setting. The unmodified floors house forty-four residents. That is too many residents to make a home. Years ago, we started exploring the idea of modifying the floors into houses for ten people. The operational impact of that was difficult because the staff were broken into smaller teams. We needed to show the organization that it could be done. So I poured an entire year of operational capital into converting the first two houses on one of our floors.

I worked to establish our "must haves" with our contractor. Each house must have three components: bedrooms that look like home, a place for people to eat together in a dining room setting, and a living room. Those are the three spaces that are imperative for a house environment. We started with the existing, figure eight shaped unit and focused on a new design that would include the three necessities I mentioned. We settled on an L shaped house that works well. In the process, we continued our commitment to opening up walls and making large living spaces as opposed to long, narrow hallways. We created spaces for natural interaction and relationship building. We have foyers between homes and a foyer in front of the elevator so that visitors do not simply walk into the residents' personal space. We installed house doors at the entrance to the residence. We have the functional areas, like office space and nursing stations, in the background.

JG: How many other floors do you plan to convert?

RP: We have converted one floor so far. We have two floors in the south building that are also functioning as two small homes each. By the end of this year, we will have converted all five floors to the small home model. We will have ten more houses physically changed by the end of 2016. We will have all of the organization operationally changed to this model by 2017.

JG: Is it less profitable to have fewer residents per floor?

RP: We were lucky because we had additional space for residents in our other locations. This organization once had four hundred and seventy-five people living here. But we moved twenty to the Penfield Green Houses. At the end of this conversion, I foresee that St. John's may serve fewer people on this campus. We are exploring the possibility of serving people in their home communities. We are researching methods to discharge people into a meaningful life back in the community. That way, the elders who do not need our in-house long-term care experience can be matched to the care that fits their situation.

JG: What is the residents' average length of stay?

RP: On average, people stay in our long-term care for about thirty-five months, or almost three years. It is not a short stay. Most people come in hoping to be rehabilitated and go back home. People want to live in their homes as long as possible. There are many options for discharge. They have the possibility of going into assisted living. You saw our independent living residences. They are set up in the village model. We have a larger building with apartments, a restaurant, and common spaces that are open to the public. Residents may have their Rotary Club meet there. Or a local yoga teacher may come and teach senior yoga. The common public and private spaces are well used. Our independent living campus also has many individual homes. The independent living residences are part of our continuum. The average age of the residents of our independent living campus is eighty-five.

Another option for elders upon discharge is to move into a shared apartment type of setting. In Rochester, this program is called a Nursing Home Without Walls Waiver. Our social work staff here at St. John's help to place discharged elders to homes that have access to the services they need. Approximately two-thirds of the people who come into St. John's stay with us through the end of their life.

JG: How do the residents pay to live here?

RP: Twenty percent of our income is through private pay. About sixty percent of our income is through Medicaid. The remaining is from long-term insurance. We would like to change those ratios to increase the number of private pay residents.

JG: Is private pay more profitable?

RP: Yes. The government reimburses this organization about one hundred and thirty dollars less a day per resident than it actually costs to take care of them. One of the reasons we are implementing the Eden Alternative and small homecare is that we think we can create a cost of care that more closely matches what the government pays. The Green Houses at Penfield operate with lower costs and provide a better quality of care. In order to realize those cost savings in our legacy building, we have to convert the floors into small homes. The home-like environment also supports the culture change for the staff. Staff act more like family members by taking responsibility for all the activities of care. The staff needs to be able to cook in the neighborhood. They need to be able to do laundry in the neighborhood. They need to be able to staff and schedule themselves in a way that meets the needs of their house. They need to make culture change without the bigger organization acting like a magnet pulling them back into the hospital routine. Culture change is more difficult when not supported by the physical environment.

JG: Will you be able to reduce costs with the Eden Alternative and Green House philosophies and models of care?

RP: Our new model uses a completely different staffing plan and a completely different cultural environment. We direct much of our resources into a workforce trained in versatility who can support all the needs of the elders. By increasing the scope of the responsibilities of the employees closest to the elders, fewer housekeeping, dining, and activity support is needed. This results in lower operation costs.

JG: How is the staffing plan different from other long-term care models? Please explain what Shahbaz means.

RP: Shahbaz is a Persian word for "royal falcon." It started with the founder of the Eden Alternative, Bill Thomas, and his commitment to moving away from any aspect of this industry that cues the staff and residents to revert back to institutionalism. The words aide and nurse connote institutional behavior. Bill Thomas is a storyteller and he created the story of the Shahbaz. It is a story of a royal falcon that serves the king, who is the elder. The falcon surveys the elder's home and kingdom and identifies risks. The falcon identifies needs. The falcon identifies what is missing from this kingdom. The falcon returns and reports to the elder on how we can redirect or how we can reinvest. That is the legend of the Shahbaz. We embrace it here to create empowered, engaged employees who have the skills that they need to make the lives of the elders vibrant. It is special, but it does take some explaining.

JG: How does the Shahbaz story translate into practice?

RP: The role of the care partners is similar to a family member caring for their mother or father. We start with the premise that working at St. John's means you are going to care for people and touch them and spiritually connect with them. You will be a part of their life beyond just pill passing and documenting. People who are in the long-term care profession to connect and to create enriching relationships come to us and say, "I want to be a part of the team." Then we train them on how to keep a house in a way that meets the regulatory standards so that we do not have infections spread. We have seen great success in our small homes. If I was a care partner to a resident who was sick, I would quickly take a bleach wipe and clean any surfaces that the resident used. If I was a nurse in a traditional facility and the resident was sick, cleaning might not be part of my job description. I may leave the cleanup for the housekeeper who might arrive three hours later. Would they know the precise areas to be extra careful about cleaning three hours later? Would another resident come into contact with the unclean areas before the housekeeper arrived? The execution of cleanliness has been remarkably different in the Green House homes using Shahbaz staff and the Eden Alternative philosophy.

JG: What other roles are Shahbaz trained to perform that differ from those of the typical nurse working in long-term care?

RP: The Shahbaz or care partners are trained to cook and serve meals by a clinical dietician and cook. The dietician offers meal support by ensuring the food is the right texture, contains the right nutritional components, and is in the right quantity. We also have a scheduling coordinator to optimize staffing efficiency, a Meaningful Life coordinator to ensure meaningful activities, a Housekeeping coordinator to ensure cleanliness standards are met, a Care coordinator to ensure clinical care is maintained, and a Team coordinator to ensure training and communication are well executed.

The first line of quality assurance is a very clearly executed coordinator role that every Shahbaz will assume. Shahbazim coordinators are responsible for certain aspects of home life. For example, if I am the coordinator, I own the responsibility for the quality and safety of the home. If my fellow Shahbaz or care partner is not emptying the trash or keeping the room tidy, I would ask, "What is happening? Do we need to change the process? Do we need retraining? Do you simply need to know that I am noticing?" If the first line of fixing the issue does not work, we bring in a nurse leader, a housekeeping leader, a social worker, a recreational therapist, or the Eden Alternative guide as a coach and leader. He or she engages the care partners to come up with a plan to identify and address the issue. This process ensures that our team is working together in a way that meets the needs of the staff and the elders. This inherent quality assurance for dining, personal care, grooming, housekeeping, and scheduling is an effective model because it requires sustainable accountability in the direct care role. I have never seen anything like this model in group homes or in long-term care. Most often in traditional care facilities, the quality assurance role rests with a leader not directly involved in caring. The Shahbazim role is special and impactful.

Care partners also make sure that there are meaningful activities happening so that the residents are involved and connecting. Care partners may read aloud, do puzzles, cook, and garden with a group of the residents.

JG: Does the role of coordinator rotate?

RP: Yes. We rotate coordinators every three months. Shahbazim know they will be the coordinator every three months. This means there is not one boss. The Shahbazim all know each other's abilities. It makes for a deep understanding of the challenges of everyone's responsibilities. Everyone walks in everyone's shoes. There is no one person who holds all the power. We have a horizontal, fluid, organizational culture that breeds employee empowerment and ownership.

JG: How do you make this culture and the required training sustainable?

RP: It has been the most difficult challenge for us here because we are a large organization with many employees. There are almost nine hundred full time and part time nursing employees at St. John's. We have three hundred and forty residents in skilled nursing. We also have over four hundred and fifty at the Meadows independent living community. We are continually training and supporting our team. We found that having our staff do a forty-hour training together has been very effective. They learn about the coordinator roles. They are able to absorb the philosophy and the principles of eradicating loneliness, hopelessness, and boredom. The training teaches the integration of the Eden Alternative philosophies into day to day operations.

The training addresses many relational components. Who

are you? How do you work? What is your personality type? What is my personality type? How do we complement each other? How could we annoy each other? What are we going to do with this information? We commit to giving each house this conversation opportunity for one week each year.

Weekly team meetings run by the team coordinator of the house are also inherent to this model. The meetings are learning circles where everyone contributes their thoughts on resolving any house issues. Staff are trained in a module of Eden Neighborhood Guide Education during one weekly meeting per month. The neighborhood guide training gives the staff tactical skills for conflict resolution, decision making, and rapport building.

JG: Are the Neighborhood Guide trainings delivered via webinar or in person?

RP: We have an Eden Alternative educator in house. Her name is Kristine Angevine. She took the Eden Alternative educator course and became a certified Eden educator. She hosts trainings for us in the various aspects of the Eden Alternative. The Eden Alternative uses the train the trainer model. Kristine is creating champions for culture change.

JG: Can you give me an example of an issue that Kristine Angevine might address?

RP: My colleague and I could be having issues working together. The staff could tell us that our discord is affecting the culture of the house in a negative way. They may hear about it from the elders or their families. These types of situations present an opportunity for team accountability. Kristine would look for methods to help my colleagues and I to work through our issues. The guide is a relational mentor. The training that the Eden Alternative teaches is a tactical approach to problem solving. It is a robust, personal growth training that has applications for all groups of staff. It helps people learn how to function as a team.

JG: How do you measure outcomes?

RP: We use a key performance report that I review weekly with each of my neighborhoods. We refer to three or four houses as a neighborhood. We track financials, clinical quality, and employee satisfaction and turnover. All of these measures have seen improvement as we moved to a small home model.

JG: How do you apply person directed care to the residents with dementia?

RP: Most residents in long-term care have some stage of dementia. Mr. J is a man who lives "in organization" with dementia. Living "in organization" means that residents at all stages of dementia and aging live together. The way that Mr. J's dementia has manifested is that he does a lot of searching. He looks for things. He explores places. He is continually busy. He was a marathon runner. He was an avid traveler. Mr. J's wife was not comfortable with him living in a typical locked unit or a unit with other people who all had similar manifestations of dementia. She found a home for Mr. J in one of our traditional neighborhoods that is soon to be converted into a small home.

Mr. J had certain habits that were somewhat startling to people. Elders like Mr. P, who is alert and oriented, would say, "Why are you touching my hair?" Some residents would wake up from a sound sleep to find Mr. J sitting in their room. We took a deep look into how we could help Mr. J become well known to the staff and the residents. We worked with him and his family to determine what he needed. Mimi DeVinney is our dementia specialist. She spent time watching Mr. J, to understand his patterns and unmet needs. Mimi found that Mr. J's unmet need was touch. Touch is a very personal activity. Mimi noticed that no one was touching him proactively. She said, "Let us try something. Let us try giving Mr. J a hug when we see him. Maybe we can provide some of the human connection he is craving."

She also coached his family. His wife was taken aback because she had not touched her husband in an intimate manner in a long time. The staff hug him whenever he wants a hug. Sometimes he will walk right by and that means he does not want a hug. Instituting hugging has stopped Mr. J from touching people in search of a physical connection. It has given him a great way to make the connection he needs. Hugging also helps the staff see him differently. He has become everyone's buddy. When I hug Mr. J, we share a connection that is positive and uplifting for us both.

We wanted to create a way for people to know Mr. J when he came into the house. We made a binder with stories about him. The book shares details and photos about him in his role as an uncle. It describes him as a professional. His wife shared her story of their life together. It includes old and new stories. The book shows Mr. J as an uncle and a husband. It reminds the reader that he was an incredible professional and a marathon runner. He is no longer scary to residents when they know details about his life. He may not be able to talk about those details because they are no longer accessible to his brain. Mr. J is now seen as a man living with dementia rather than as a stranger continually strolling around.

Identity is an important component of the Eden Alternative Domains of Well-being. We strive to understand the person's history and unmet needs. This understanding informs us how to best connect to each other. Meeting needs and connecting to each other is the foundation of well-being.

JG: How many people that you care for have dementia?

RP: Eighty-five percent of the four hundred and fifty residents here at the 150 Highland Avenue residence are living with some form of dementia. There are two floors with no exit available to the residents. We have approximately sixty residents on those floors.

JG: Will you convert those floors into small houses also?

RP: Absolutely. We cannot convert them quickly enough.

JG: Are you converting the floors because the small home supports better dementia care?

RP: Yes. A simple example is when a resident is looking for something, he or she can look all around, they can go into the kitchen and the living room, they can look through the bookshelves and cupboards. There are no off limits areas. The residents are much more likely to find what they are searching for. Sometimes residents cannot communicate their need to find something with us. Small homes are an environment wherein they can search and search. Al Power, the international educator of culture change in long-term care and an Eden Alternative board member, regularly says, "Policies that are good for people with dementia are almost always good for everyone." I agree. We all need to be known and understood. We all need to feel connected. We all need to belong and to have some level of independence. Good dementia care is good elder care and vice versa.

We do not segregate people by their diagnoses. Instead, we create opportunities for elders who are alert and oriented to interact with those who have different challenges. That has worked out well for us.

JG: Other than what you have already discussed, what are your thoughts on person directed care in the long-term care setting?

RP: Maintaining person directed care is sometimes difficult due to specific regulations. Regulations only support activities that pose no risk to the residents. If a resident wants to smoke a cigarette on our smoke free campus, our organization tries to create a plan for him or her to go off campus to smoke. The Department of Health scrutinizes every aspect of that plan. It is difficult for them to understand how an organization could support a smoke free campus and yet help people smoke if they wish. The regulations are based on risk aversion.

JG: Are there regulatory issues with your practice of allowing residents full use of the kitchens and the ability to eat whatever and whenever they wish?

RP: We communicate the details of our process of keeping the kitchen safe and sanitary to regulatory agencies. A dedicated leader of person directedness does not ever say, "No, we cannot do that." The leader says, "Yes. How do we do that? What policies do we need to put in place? What training do we need to put in place? What quality measures do we need to put in place?" It takes dedication and hard work, but it is worth it.

JG: Do you have to remain adaptive and innovative in order to meet each resident's need?

RP: That is why the Shahbazim model is so effective. Innova-tion should happen right there in the house. It should not be my or any other administrator's policy. We support an operational structure that allows for innovation and quality assurance from the staff, without blanket policies from the administration. We have had some struggles, but we have had significant change and success.

JG: Can you share an example?

RP: A resident in one of our houses has a family member who likes to go into the kitchen and make a sandwich for their parent and themselves. The first reaction of staff was to prohibit family: "No. My kitchen, my rules." Their reaction was based on concern for rules and safety. We had to rethink our initial response. It is not our kitchen. It is their mom's kitchen. If I walk into my mom's kitchen, I can go into the refrigerator and take whatever I want. I might make a sandwich for her. The staff and I sat down and worked through all the issues surrounding this situation. We decided to give that family member her own shelf. We taught her to date the food that she stores on her shelf. She has to replace the food regularly to meet the safety requirements. The food coordinator will also make sure the family member's shelf is stocked.

In another house, there might be an elder who wants his or her own food. It is necessary to have a dining leader. Our chief dietician will coach the care team to be creative. There cannot be a "no" as a response. We expect the Shahbaz team to be innovative and responsive. With that expectation comes our responsibility, as management, to create an organizational environment where people feel supported and safe to innovate. This is beginning to come to fruition within our Penfield residences. It took us about eighteen months before we witnessed the changes. I imagine it will take the houses here at Highland Avenue eighteen months to two years. Culture change takes time.

JG: Is it the job of the Shahbazim to organize as much as they can around the personality and lifestyle of the resident?

RP: Yes. The resident might have a better idea of how we can do things differently. Each resident needs different care and connections. I bring my own cultural nuances to my life here. Each person who moves into one of our residences does the same. We are forcing residents to live with people who have very different life stories. Our job at St. John's is to allow the staff to enable residents to live how they want to live. We do this to the extent that the choice is safe and possible.

JG: In what aspects, other than home design, do you involve the residents' input?

RP: We seek resident input on staff selection. They sit through the interview. Our resident council reviews our finances each quarter. Residents lead staffing ratio choices. The tricky part with elder input is creating the reason for changes that ensure the staff buy in. We must enable staff to know that we can operate a long-term care residence in a very different cultural structure. We have experienced some challenges with change. Changing a system means you have to admit it is not working optimally. In some situations, leadership has to step in and make it clear that the new direction and culture change is not optional.

JG: Is the culture change you are referring to the change from a legacy industrial type of culture to one based on the Eden Alternative principles?

RP: Yes.

JG: Please share a little bit more about the culture change.

RP: I'll give you an example. We had an elder who moved while her room was being renovated. She lives with dementia. She became comfortable in her temporary room and did not want to move into the room we had prepared for her. The staff from her original house knew her and loved her. They were attached and wanted her back. They said, "She cannot make that decision. She will say yes to anything. We need her back. We love her." We had four different people meet with the resident to be sure. In the end, she did not want to move again. That was absolutely within her right. We were not asking her to make a life or death decision. We may have been somewhat challenged by the old paternalistic culture of thinking that we know what is best.

But we took the time to understand her wishes. That resident is happy. She is connected. She has a new friend.

JG: How has your staff taken to the new Shahbaz concept of care?

RP: I estimate that ninety percent of our team is thrilled with this conversion once they understand and become a part of the new paradigm. After the fear of change and the confusion subside, the staff realize the benefit of working as a team and caring for residents as a family member would. The model eventually makes sense to the staff.

There are some people who fit better in a hospital type of care model. They find a way to self-select out. The ones who stay are the people who support the mission of person directed care. They are here because they want more time with the elders and they see that happening with the new culture. They are the people who are here because they want to take care of the whole person. The care partners receive meaningful relationships in return. They are able to share who they are in a different way. The ninety percent of my staff who have gone through this transition has grown to love the new culture.

JG: Has your transition to the Eden Alternative and Green House model made life as a caregiver less stressful or depressing?

RP: Yes. We have realized impressive results in caregiver burnout and turnover because of our conversion to the Eden Alternative and small house long-term care model.

JG: Do you think this model of care might entice more medical students into the field of geriatrics?

RP: I hope so. Geriatrics is an emotional practice because you are often saying goodbye. It is an emotional practice because you have the family dynamic component. Family members who often live far away will try to micromanage their parent's healthcare. Another big barrier is that nursing homes and geriatricians are targeted daily by our legal system. Tort law needs to be reined in because the exposure of those caring for the elderly is large.

I hope that this model will speak to physicians. I have met many people who are in school now or just coming out into their fellowships who understand that our care culture creates a better life experience. What happens, though, is that they end up working in an existing health system and they do not have the time, the resources, the technology, or the organizational support to live the culture change. St. John's is special. Geriatricians need an environment that supports innovation and growth. Hopefully we can share our proof that this model drives improved outcomes for the business, staff, and residents. Our encouraging outcomes, population aging, and the unsustainable long-term care need will all drive system change.

JG: Please tell me about your Brickstone campus.

RP: Brickstone is an independent living community built around the village square concept. It is organized around the importance of community. We maintain a commitment to keeping the residents involved and not isolated. The residents stay engaged. The community is filled with common spaces. The village square concept brings elders and the public community together in restaurants, boutiques, stores, and meeting halls. It is a senior housing model that is geared to fifty-five and older, but most of our residents are over seventy-five. Brickstone is more of an upscale model that caters to people with slightly higher income levels. We charge month to month and the rents are at or just above market value. Rents range from one to three thousand dollars per month. Residents do not have to pay any buy-in. And there is no obligation for them to stay. We have events at Brickstone also. We had a wedding for the granddaughter of one of the residents. We also have many community groups that use the common spaces regularly. They host the local Rotary. The Parkinson's Foundation has monthly meetings there. We have a collaborative relationship with the community and we allow community groups to hold their meetings on the campus.

JG: Are the residents welcome at those meetings?

RP: Yes, the residents are welcome. Often the residents generate the connections because they belong to the groups. We have built many community partnerships.

We have yoga classes that are cosponsored by St. John's and MVP, a local health insurance provider. We have brought in programming from the Jewish Community Center. In January, we showed the movie *Advanced Style*, which is based on a New York City blog. We invited the community at large and hosted a fashion consultant to present. The public-private collaborations we create make for an active and engaging campus.

We strive to not just make sure elders can age in community with other elders, but to make sure that Brickstone is a place that attracts younger generations. They want to go hang out where their grandmother lives. They want to go to Brickstone because they have great functions, stores, restaurants, exercise classes, courses, and boutiques. We brought in local organic farmers to hold a fair and started a community supported agriculture program where people can join to receive seasonal fruits and vegetables. We hosted the Holistic Approach Fair. The Northstar Healthcare Business Academy has leaders who come and speak.

JG: Do the residents of Brickstone by St. John's have input into the operations?

RP: Yes. Elder input begins the first day of independent living and continues on when the residents are transferred into our skilled nursing facilities. Paul Bartlett, the Vice President of Senior Housing, hosts a coffee chat at both Brickstone and the Meadows every week. Residents discuss any number of things, such as whether the windows are washed. It is an open forum. It keeps the residents involved and engaged in the community.

JG: Do many residents in independent living eventually move into your long-term care facilities?

RP: Yes. Many residents transfer from independent living or rehabilitation to skilled care. Residents are interested in experiencing the continuum of care with the same culture of inclusion. It is familiar and gives them peace of mind. Once you are part of the St. John's family we will take care of you. That is the message.

JG: Do you involve children and animals in your communities?

RP: Yes. Including animals, plants, and children is part of Bill and Jude Thomas's Eden Alternative model.

We established a children's day care center, Generations, on the campus of St. John's Home in 2002. It is a unique endeavor that facilitates continued intergenerational connections. The children visit the residents regularly. We also have special events to include the children. One of those events is "plant pals," where children and elders partner to plant and cultivate our onsite Trinity Garden.

We have a dog named Lexi who lives in one of our Green House residences in the Penfield neighborhood. We adopted her about a year ago. She is a five-and-a-half-year-old, seventy-pound Labrador Mastiff mix. She brings a lot of joy to the residents. The elders consider her to be part of their family.

JG: Do providers from other countries come here to learn from you?

RP: Yes. There are many curious innovators who want to learn from us. In the last month, we hosted someone from Germany, and two people from different entities in New Zealand. We have also hosted people from Switzerland and Singapore.

People are starting to take notice. We had quite a few visitors who are in the Canadian market and are looking to create something different within their national healthcare system. They are taken with our Green Houses at Penfield. They are curious to learn how the small home model can transfer into an existing home or legacy structure. They are exploring how the transfer can be accomplished with relatively few resources. Someday we hope to be a little more resource rich. At this time, we are not cash rich or significantly endowed. But we were able to implement the Eden Alternative and Green House models. Lower finances are not a barrier to this sort of change.

JG: Has your bottom line suffered from the remodel and culture overhaul?

RP: No. We have only grown our business through these changes.

JG: Profitability has grown?

RP: Profitability and quality. They go hand in hand. What we have seen in small homes is a much better quality with much more ability to be profitable.

JG: Is the profitability increasing because insurers and the Centers for Medicaid and Medicare see the quality and cost improvement?

RP: No. We are also not charging more. Our increased profits are realized because of better efficiency and expense reduction. People are willing to pay us privately because of our reputation for quality.

JG: At what percentage is your current occupancy?

RP: We are ninety-five percent occupied.

JG: What percentage of your occupants pay privately?

RP: Eighteen percent. Private payers are the lifeblood of our model. We are able to remain sustainable while caring for people who need Medicaid by reducing overall cost and improving staff retention. If you provide the best quality living, you rarely have empty rooms. We had a strong brand when we began. Implementing the Eden Alternative and Green House models have only strengthened our brand.

JG: Can other countries emulate this model?

RP: I think the Eden Alternative has great prototypes to train people. People would have to participate in culture training and make a culture shift in their organization. That is where they would start. Then they would continue the training and receive support with Eden Alternative people.

Leadership is key. If you do not have a leader who believes in creating a home that meets each individual elder's needs, it will not work. Traditional fear-based leadership cannot facilitate the culture of the Eden Alternative.

JG: You obviously have a great leader and you have become one yourself. How important is the support of the board in your transformation?

RP: It is instrumental. Our leadership started with the board. Charlie worked with the board and cultivated their support. The board is now our number one supporter. They are all leaders in this new culture of care and inclusion.

JG: Thank you for this insightful and interesting interview.

RP: Thank you for coming to Rochester. You are welcome back at any time.

— END OF INTERVIEW —

Dementia Beyond Disease

An interview with **Allen Power**

About Allen Power

Allen Power, M.D. is a board certified internist and geriatrician, a clinical associate professor of medicine at the University of Rochester, and a Fellow of the American College of Physicians and the American Society for Internal Medicine. Dr. Power is a certified Eden Alternative Educator, a member of the Eden Alternative board of directors, and an international educator on transformational models of care for older adults, particularly those living with changing cognitive abilities.

Dr. Power's book *Dementia Beyond Drugs: Changing the Culture of Care* won a 2010 Book of the Year Award from the *American Journal of Nursing*, a Merit Award from the 2011 National Mature Media Awards, and was listed as a "must have" title in *Doody's Core Titles* list for 2013. He has co-produced two DVDs with Dr. Richard Taylor and Brilliant Image Productions: *Living with Dementia* and *20 Questions, 100 Answers, 6 Perspectives*. Dr. Power was interviewed for the film *Alive Inside*, winner of the Audience Award for Best US Documentary at the 2014 Sundance Film Festival. His two-day Eden Alternative course, *Dementia Beyond Drugs*, has been taught in nine states and five countries.

Dr. Power was awarded a Bellagio Residency in Italy in 2012 by the Rockefeller Foundation, where he worked with Dr. Emi Kiyota on developing guidelines for sustainable communities that embrace people of

all ages and abilities. He is a consultant for Dr. Kiyota's non-profit orga-
nization Ibasho, as well as a member of the Leadership Council for the
Dementia Action Alliance, and serves in an advisory capacity for the
Music and Memory project, Dementia Care Australia, and the South
Africa Care Forum.

Dr. Power recorded introductory material for the new Centers for
Medicare and Medicaid Services educational package, "Hand in
Hand," designed to help hands-on staff better care for people living
with dementia. He has served in an advisory capacity with the Centers
for Medicare and Medicaid Services and worked with the National
Dementia Initiative to produce a white paper about new approaches to
dementia for the US Senate Special Committee on Aging.

Dr. Power is a featured contributor to Eden Founder Dr. Bill Thomas's
weblog at www.changingaging.org. He has been interviewed by the
BBC, the *New York Times*, the *Washington Post*, the *Los Angeles Times*,
the *Wall Street Journal*, the *New Yorker*, Singapore's *Straits Times*, ABC
Radio (Australia), WHYY radio, WXXI radio, many other publications
and radio shows, and for the book *Old Age in a New Age: The Promise
of Transformative Nursing Homes* by Beth Baker.

Dr. Power is also a trained musician and songwriter with three record-
ings, including *Life Worth Living: A Celebration of Elders and Those
Who Care for Them*. His songs have been recorded by several artists
and performed on three continents. Peter, Paul, and Mary performed
his song of elder autonomy, "If You Don't Mind," and Walter Cronkite
used his song "I'll Love You Forever" in a 1995 Discovery Channel profile of American families.

INTERVIEW

Jean Galiana (JG): Please share the journey that led you to
becoming an author and speaker about dementia.

Allen Power (AP): I started as a geriatrician in private practice as an internist. After about seven years of working as an
internist I became a little burned out. I was drawn into long

term care and worked in a large nursing home complex. Over time and mostly due to the Eden Alternative, I discovered the culture change movement that was beginning to form. The nursing home where I was practicing did not want to embrace culture change, so I moved to St. John's Home in Rochester, where I worked for almost fourteen years. I was always concerned with the use of antipsychotic medications and similar drugs in people with dementia. I tried not to use them whenever possible. I continually spoke out against them and challenged coworkers to find other solutions. I received a lot of pushback, as you can imagine. This was well before anyone was talking about the high usage of these medicines.

It remained a challenge for me because I had a view of culture change with a bigger vision than I could yet articulate. I did not completely understand it myself. I often say, "when you do not understand a subject as well as you would like, the best thing to do is write a book about it." That belief is what led me to write my first book, *Dementia Beyond Drugs*. It took me three years to write it. The book was my attempt to explain what was wrong with only using medications when people are stressed. I knew that we needed to find new ways to interact with people with dementia that challenged the existing view of dementia care. I also delved into some of the transformational principles of culture change to care for people living with memory challenges. This type of person centered care is based in the work of Tom Kitwood, the psychologist from the United Kingdom. He introduced person centered thinking approximately twenty years ago. My book is the first person centered dementia care guide written by a medical doctor. I received some nice reviews after its publication. Not much else happened for a couple of years until the Centers for Medicare and Medicaid Services began to focus on reducing the use of antipsychotic medications. More and more evidence came out against the overmedication of people with dementia in long term living. My book gained in popularity, and I was regularly asked to speak and to consult. I migrated out of working in the medical setting and became a culture change specialist at St. John's Home, traveling around to speaking engagements. Three years ago, I made the shift to full time speaker and consultant. That is a long way from where I started back in private practice. Life takes us to surprising places sometimes.

JG: Please describe your book, *Dementia Beyond Drugs*.

AP: *Dementia Beyond Drugs* challenged the entire paradigm of dementia. It presented different ways to conceptualize living with dementia and proposed better options to transform our approach to care. My second book, *Dementia Beyond Disease*, was meant to further the thoughts of the first, but I was not really sure what to write about. I had not been practicing at that point, so I did not have many more of my own stories to tell. I decided to tell stories of best practice that I witnessed during my travels. I also decided to focus on a model of well-being that a handful of culture change specialists had designed. I thought it would be nice to write a book that examines dementia through the lens of the seven Eden Alternative Domains of Well-being. I originally planned it as an addendum to my first book, but it turned out to be forty pages longer. That is how the second book originated. It led me to create a strengths based approach to people with dementia, where instead of just trying to mitigate problems, you are actually enhancing well-being proactively. The strengths based approach has enabled care partners to successfully address certain challenges that were insurmountable before. It really opened the door to new ways of thinking.

After *Dementia Beyond Disease* had been out for two years, my publisher came back to me and said, "The first book is still selling well. I think it is time to come up with a second edition and update it." I did not want to rewrite my second book into my first. When it came to revising the first book, I tried to keep the same format, even though my view of dementia had moved a little bit. I kept the format and updated some of the stories. The main thing I changed was the language. I thought my language was enlightened when I wrote the first book. Six years later I looked at it and cringed, so I changed a lot of wording and updated some of my terminology. That second edition came out in October 2016.

Then, as things often happen, my second book went to a reprinting at the same time. The publishers told me that they were not going to print a second edition but wanted me to read it through for words I thought could be replaced by better words and other minor changes. When I read what I had written about the dedicated staff initiative my friends implemented at Arcare in Australia, I realized that there were many new outcomes they had tracked since the book was published. I wanted to add those along with a couple of quotes. Because my new book was coming out as a new edition with a new copyright date, we decided to release the second book as a revised edition. It is essentially the same book.

JG: Please discuss the transformational principles you mentioned.

AP: The Eden Alternative informs much of my work, but I also work with the Green House Project and the Pioneer Network. There are many people I work with who are involved with culture change. In the case of dementia, I look at transforming three aspects. Personal transformation consists of the intrapersonal—which is changing the way we see dementia, changing how we view people living with dementia, and understanding their needs—and the interpersonal dimension—which is changing the way we communicate with those living with dementia. That comprises one aspect of transformation. A second is the physical living environment. Does it support people who live with dementia or does it not? We examine what policies and practices help or hinder well-being for people with dementia, including medical and physical restraints and alarms. We also examine how homey and warm the setting is.

The third aspect, which I consider the lynchpin, is the operational transformation. As I say in the book, neither a holistic mindset nor a beautiful building will matter if you do not change day to day operations. This includes how decisions are made and how staff interacts with the residents. In the case of community based living, it includes how family members are adjusting to the rhythms and needs of the person. Sundowning is a result of forcing people to conform to our rhythms. That is why it happens in the home as well as in the long-term living homes. Family care is challenging because it is difficult for one person to meet another's needs twenty-four hours a day. Caregivers need to sleep and run errands. It is very hard to individualize care around the rhythms of someone. Long-term living residences often have the goal of person directed culture, but they do not adapt to the personal rhythms of eating, sleeping, toilet use, and bathing. Providers build nice buildings but do not make the important cultural shift necessary to achieve person directed lifestyles for their residents.

JG: You mentioned sundowning and the relationship to neglecting personal rhythms. Have you witnessed light adjustments that also lead to a decreased incidence of sundowning?

AP: There is no question that we all need cues. If you live in a place like I do with little light for six months a year, you see many people who experience seasonal depression. There is no question sunlight is important to people. I think that lighting could be helpful, but to affect circadian rhythms, the light must be strong. I am not sure if just having indoor incandescent lights that dim or brighten would be useful.

With Seasonal Affective Disorder, you need to shine a bright lamp about twelve to eighteen inches from your face first thing in the morning for a half hour to an hour. To me, the answer is to bring people outdoors. Even on a cloudy day, the sun is still much brighter and broader in spectrum than anything available indoors. Why not have people go out and sit or build a snowman like they do at the Green Houses at St. John's in Rochester?

JG: They have residents build snowmen at St. John's Home?

AP: Yes. All it takes is fifteen minutes of good sunlight to make a big difference. You can do other things like design with skylights and big windows and things that bring natural light into the environment also. Organizing practices around the residents' changing rhythms reduces or eliminates sundowning most effectively. The best option is to support the changing rhythms of the residents and create an environment that is flexible enough to accommodate those rhythms as much as possible. A good example of creating opportunities that honor the rhythms of the resident can be found at Hebrew Home of Riverdale. Residents who are up at night can go to their nightclub. Rather than requiring people to go to bed at a set hour, they offer other options. Normal aging causes changes in our sleep architecture and sleep duration that are difficult to fix with sleeping pills. The drugs tend to do more harm than good. The goal of person directed living is working around the rhythms of the residents and not trying to force ours on them.

JG: Does it require more staff to adjust to the personal rhythms of the residents?

AP: This is why I emphasize the third part the operational transformation. It may appear that person directed culture would require more staff, but it requires fewer than the traditional siloed culture that is built upon a hierarchical environment model. Fewer staff are needed when you remove silos and create flexibility with dedicated staffing. A dedicated staff knows each resident so deeply that the care is easier and the connection more fluid. The practice of rotating staff assignments means the roster changes, the order in which you do things changes, the personalities you deal with change, and the way you interact with your coworkers changes because you are interacting with different people who do things differently. Rotating staff adds many layers of inefficiency. It sounds convenient but it is not. The institutional model is not efficient. I am one of the people who has been guilty of spreading the myth that institutions have thrived because they favor efficiency over people. The truth is that there is nothing efficient about institutions.

JG: Please give an example of best practice in dedicated staff assignments.

AP: Daniella Greenwood of Arcare in Australia led her team to dedicated staff assignments. They made the shift because the residents and their families who participated in a survey asked for improved connections and continuous relationships. If you believe in consumer directed care, then you give the customer what they want. They had no idea of the profound health outcomes the choice would produce. Those things were icing on the cake. Any good business will adapt itself around the needs of people.

JG: Did their shift from rotated staff to dedicated staff assignments take Arcare a long time?

AP: It took them six weeks in their first community before they could claim that the staff was spending more time with the elders and were also able to complete their tasks. The entire process was rolled out sequentially over their twenty-seven communities over a three-year period.

JG: What outcomes did moving to a dedicated staff assignment produce at Arcare?

AP: The results from one early adopting community of thirty-eight residents saw a sixty-nine percent decrease in chest infections, ninety percent decrease in pressure injuries, and five percent increase in family satisfaction. They have many other impressive outcomes for the residents, the family members, and the team members as well, such as increased satisfaction and decreased turnover.

JG: The concept seems simple.

AP: Yes, but change is difficult. To change an organizational culture, you must engage everyone. Most systems reinforce the old industrialized ways of thinking and acting. An example that I added to the new edition of *Dementia Beyond Disease* is that in New York State, insurers pay a per bed premium to anyone who has a nursing home with more than three hundred beds. They are incentivizing the warehousing of older people by building these huge institutional buildings. In order to create a person directed culture, the organizations will have to adapt to a badly built environment. These large buildings offer little access to the outdoors. They also have long clinical hallways that create too much distance between residents and common areas. There is inefficiency getting from one resident's room to another.

JG: When was that policy enacted?

AP: In the 1960s and 1970s. The policy presented me with a wonderful opportunity to learn. Most small homes have a doctor who comes once or twice a month. St. John's Home was so large that it gave me the ability to be a full time doctor in a nursing home community. I was there every day getting to know the staff and residents and working on culture change. As a physician, I was able to deeply understand culture change. However, warehousing older adults is not the best way to care for people.

JG: Do you have an opinion about whether staff should or should not wear uniforms?

AP: Uniforms reinforce the medical model. We try to create a home, particularly for people who may be somewhat confused about what home is. They need all the cues we can give them. Regular clothes are as much a physical cue as a nice living room. Uniforms send two messages. One is the message of power and control. Uniforms represent power, whether it is the uniform of a police officer, a member of the military, a nurse, or a doctor. The other message of uniforms in long-term care is, you are here because you are sick. This tends to promote dependency among residents. You sit back and become a patient when you see everyone walking around in uniforms. We have witnessed that response to uniforms. I have heard stories of communities where they see the residents becoming much more independent and doing more for themselves when the staff change from wearing uniforms to wearing street clothes. Providers who do not use uniforms give the employees a clothing budget. Some people worry whether the residents will know who the care partners are. St. John's is a leading example with regard to person directed care without uniforms.

JG: I was there and at first I could not tell whether they were staff or family.

AP: The interesting thing is that the residents do know who the care partners are because the staff does not rotate. They are there every day. The relationships between the care partners and the residents are close and loving. You do not see people trying to get out the front door. You do not see people walking into each other's rooms. Many dementia related behaviors are triggered by the environment. They are triggered when we

180

create confusion. It stems from a desire to find something that the care partners are not providing. It is possible to cure these things with the culture of care partnership.

JG: Please tell me about your speaking tour.

AP: I travel around the world speaking about dementia. I updated my geriatrician certification exam a couple of years ago, but my talks are mostly nonmedical. My talks and books are mostly nonscientific. I made that choice intentionally for a couple of reasons. Doctors use a lot of technical language. To me that is another entrapment of power. If you can baffle people with the technical talk, they have to defer to what you say. I am determined to communicate a model that is easily understood and makes sense. We need a model that people can apply to all residences, no matter what form of dementia or other challenges their residents face. If someone is teaching an approach to dementia that requires a certified nursing assistant to know that a resident has a particular type and stage of dementia before they can respond, the care model is worthless. That is what I love about truly person directed care: it is universal. It is universal across cultures, ethnicities, and abilities.

I also consult with organizations to help them understand how to fully operationalize person directed long-term living. I consult often with Schlegel Villages in Canada. The Research Institute for Aging partnered with Schlegel Villages to research and measure outcomes of their relational living model.

JG: In one of your talks you mentioned the existential, spiritual experience of dementia. Please describe what you mean.

AP: In Christine Bryden's first book, *Who Will I Be When I Die?*, she wrote about how people go through existential questions when they are struck with a new illness. The diagnosis makes them think about their mortality and their abilities. In *Dementia Beyond Disease*, I wrote about how people who lose easy access to memories or to language sometimes become hyper-attuned to other senses such as non-verbal communications. People living with dementia can view things in symbolic or metaphorical ways instead of literally. We need to understand this to be able to hone our communication skills. We are communicating with our whole bodies and our tone of voice.

JG: What are your thoughts about touch for those living with dementia?

AP: When you cannot connect through language or reminiscence, touch is a way of connecting that is powerful. It is powerful from infancy. There have been many studies about the need of touch for children to develop normally. We know how important touch is throughout life. Touch stimulates other pathways in the brain that continue to function. There is a massage therapist who has worked at St. John's Home who has seen massage free people's ability to speak and remember after a session. There are many ways to stimulate people in areas where their brain can still connect. Learning which methods work for each individual and applying them is a perfect example of person directed care partnering. Music also has the power to find its way into a brain that may have some challenges.

JG: Would you discuss your blog series, *The Hidden Restraint?*

AP: We tend to view the idea of safety and security through a narrow lens. It is a lens of physical safety. It is the litigious lens of preventing the worst-case scenario. I do not want to minimize anyone being hurt, but we are only seeing one side of the security issue. I define security as supporting both emotional and psychological security. Many restraints, including locked doors, have the opposite effect. They actually make people much less secure because they cannot get out and cannot move freely. They feel trapped and often also feel that they need to get away from something. As a result, we are trading one kind of safety for another kind of security and, in many cases, making people feel worse instead of better. Is the locked door really helping the residents or the providers?

Bill Thomas speaks about the downside risk of surplus safety. Risk is not good or bad. Risk is just the chance that something will turn out differently than planned. Different can be better. If you go outside, you might fall . . . or you might sleep better. You also might not experience sundowning. You might have better strength and balance. You might be less likely to take a swing at somebody when they get in your space. There is no way to enable quality of life and eliminate all risk. We have to continually negotiate risk. That is what I write about in *The Hidden Restraint* blog. If you have people wanting to leave all the time, then before you unlock the doors you must eliminate all of the stressors that make them want to leave. That is the important place to start.

In the book, I tell stories about providers who were successful at unlocking the doors. I have a great story from Heather Luth at Schlegel Villages in Ontario. They had a gentleman who was constantly at the door. It is a perfect example, because he was stressed every day. He was either medicated or about to be medicated because he was at the door trying to get out. He said, "I just want to sit outside. I want to get some fresh air and see people." They negotiated and decided with staff to give him the key code. When I went to visit the home a few months ago, the resident was greeting visitors at the door and pushing the code to let them in. When I left, he was sitting outside on the bench and watching people come and go. Heather said that in the four years since they have done this, he has actually caught the bus three times. People have had to bring him back. Fortunately, he had no injury, but three days of getting away versus four years of daily pounding on the door and being medicated with dangerous drugs is a perfect example of risk verses quality of life.

Those are the concepts a provider must balance. Which is better? Which is worse? There is no zero risk. Bill Thomas says that the only risk in a human environment is a coffin. We have to understand that for every person who leaves the home there are hundreds of people who are being put on antipsychotics, who are distressed and traumatized every single day behind a locked door. They are withdrawing and giving up on life. That never makes the news. We have to balance those two. You cannot just help that one person and damage the other hundred.

JG: In balancing risk and quality, should the providers involve the wishes of the family and the resident?

AP: Providers must involve everyone in the care circle, including everyone in touch with the resident and their family. We all must explore people's values and understand what their tolerance for risk is, because each individual has a different risk tolerance. Some residents would say, "I do not want anything bad to happen to me, I just want some fresh air from time to time." Other people may say, "I do not care if I get run over by a truck tomorrow. I have to be able to go outside."

Everyone needs to be brought to the decision making table, including management, staff, family, and the resident. The resident must be kept in the loop, no matter their cognitive abilities. No one should be surprised by not being informed of the plan. This is where lawsuits arise. As a practicing doctor, I have gone to medical malpractice seminars for years. Most lawsuits come from poor communication, not from true malpractice. If a provider does not communicate, they are setting themselves up for trouble because people need to understand why the provider makes the choices they do. On the surface it may not make sense. It is also important to document all conversations for the regulators. Legally, if it is not written in the chart, it never happened. I have asked many regulators, and they have told me that they do not expect that nothing bad will ever happen in a nursing home. They just need to know that there is a valid thought process in the planning and operations.

JG: Is there a fine balance between mitigating risk and facilitating well-being?

AP: We try to prevent the one terrible thing from happening, but in doing so, we cause daily distress, which results in over-medication. In this scenario, well-being needs are completely ignored and the aspect of meaningful life is nonexistent. This is not because providers are bad people. Their system is focused on tasks and excess surplus safety while well-being and quality of life are ignored.

JG: Do restraints make a person safer?

AP: That is a good question. I used to talk about how restraints create safety at the expense of well-being. Studies show that they were not even creating safety. With restraints, people are more likely to be injured and more likely to have serious falls when they were allowed to stand than those who were not. Restraints were making people feel less emotionally secure and less safe. Once again, one has to ask the question: Can you even make that argument for locked doors? I do not know whether you can go that far, but if people are becoming distressed and falling down because they are constantly at the door, you can make the argument that locked doors create less physical safety as well as more emotional insecurity.

JG: Do you see a trend for unlocking doors?

AP: Not yet. That is why I maintain such a vigorous speaking calendar. Some organizations, like the St. John's Green House homes, do not lock the doors. They are out there on the fringe. Unfortunately, some of the brightest leaders are waiting for a study to prove that unlocking the doors is morally the right thing to do. Other providers have just unlocked the doors because they know it is the right thing to do. They are using their moral compass to direct their thinking. This is a personal challenge for me because I have never been a confrontational person by nature. If anything, I am just the opposite. As I try to construct an ethos around dementia that works, I start noticing the practices that contradict the philosophy. I have two choices: either be a hypocrite or speak up. The practice of locking people in is one of those areas. If you truly care about well-being, autonomy, and security, you have to understand that locking doors is not helping. It is making things worse.

JG: Have there been studies regarding chemical and physical restraints and safety?

AP: Yes. They proved that restraints increase the risk of serious injuries, increase emotional distress, and increase many other types of morbidity such as bedsores, incontinence, and muscle wasting. Those studies drove the big push by the government and most of the providers to end the use of restraints. Surprisingly, there are still a few organizations that have not made the change.

JG: Does the same apply to chemical restraints such as antipsychotic medications?

AP: Yes. People will ask me, "What about people with dual diagnoses such as dementia and lifelong schizophrenia? We do not really feel we can stop their antipsychotic." That is acceptable because the person has another condition. Possibly they cannot stop using an antipsychotic medication, but the person with the duel diagnosis still needs well-being. If you are showering them and they hit you, it may not be due to their schizophrenia. The reason may be where, how, or when you are showering them. The method or time of showering may challenge their autonomy or security. Maybe the staff rotates and the person assisting in the shower is a stranger. Just because a person has another diagnosis does not mean person directed commitment by the providers is unimportant. I also emphasize that autonomy is important with staff and family members. If you do not have autonomy or meaning in your job, how are you going to bring it to anyone else?

JG: Do you mean well-being for the staff?

AP: Exactly. I think that lack of well-being is a key contributor to burnout and caregiver turnover. New employees mean new people around the residents, and added training costs to the organization.

JG: What would you say to a nursing home administrator who is hesitant to desegregate those living with dementia from the rest of the community?

AP: The most important factors to maintaining a successful desegregated community are education, education, and education. The antidote to any kind of fear or concern or improper interaction is to educate people. There is too much stigma around dementia. There is so much fear that people do not how to respond and react to someone who has difficulty thinking. Providers need to learn the many good evidence based communication techniques. All the instruction we give to staff members should also be given to the other residents and to family members.

Why, when someone has a memory challenge, are they treated differently? When I was with St. John's Home, we had residents who did not have dementia provide companionship to people who did. It gave the residents who were helping a purpose. It also created a community connection for the person who was living with dementia, rather than ostracizing them for being different. It is a great benefit to the whole community.

It boils down to the need for education and modeling, which leads to the crucial aspect of relationship and connection. When someone who has been living in a neighborhood, a nursing home, or assisted living for a long time develops dementia, their neighbors who know them almost always accept them. When a new person living with dementia moves into a community, the fear and resistance arise. I have seen these dynamics over and over again. Relationship is the key. This is where the importance of modeling enters the scene. Providers need to educate the staff and the community about the new resident. The resident is no longer able to tell their own story, but their families can offer insights and details. The residents and staff can meet the family and learn about the life, hobbies, and unique characteristics of the newcomer. Was he a doctor? If so, possibly he should be referred to as doctor. Was she a professor? Maybe we should use professor before her name. This puts the person in front of the challenges. If you share the whole person with their neighbors, that helps decrease the fear of unfamiliarity as well.

JG: Does segregating those living with dementia contribute to the stigma?

AP: People living with dementia should be given the respect and dignified attention that they deserve. In many ways, we are reinforcing those stigmas and fears by locking up people whose brains have changed. That sends the message to the other residents that they are right and people with dementia are dangerous or odd and do not belong around them. People with dementia deserve for us to see them for who they are beyond their limitations. If you start having trouble remembering, would you like us to take you away from your friends because we do not want you around anymore? How would you feel? The best providers to those living with dementia understand that it is about preserving people's humanity as much as possible. If you were the administrator, what would you say to angry residents and family members who told you that they do not want any African American or Jewish people on the unit? You would tell them that those are not your beliefs and that thinking does not align with the mission of your organization. It is the same for someone living with dementia, if you truly support inclusive communities. The big irony is that everyone is talking about dementia friendly communities, which are inclusive communities, yet the only dementia unfriendly sector now is long-term care. I do not understand why long-term care providers seem to be giving up. Providers continue to lock people in. Challenging that practice would be a great initiative for life plan communities around the world.

JG: Do you meet with resistance when you advocate for desegregated living?

AP: Sometimes. This is a new concept, so it is understandable to a degree. It is mainly about appealing to our sense of humanity. I remember when we first built our Green Houses. We planned to move the homes off campus and into a neighborhood. Charlie Runyon, our CEO, passed the idea by the town supervisor, who loved it, but he was afraid that the neighborhood council would not. We were faced with the "not in my backyard" thinking that many people have about group homes. In response, Charlie took the impressive Green House promotional video, an urn of coffee, and a basket of homemade cookies to the neighborhood association. After that day, the neighborhood residents were enthusiastic and even offered to visit the residents and bring their dogs over. One offered to cook Thanksgiving dinner. Sometimes we sell people short. People want to be good. They want to help. When we emphasize that we all want to be accepted, no matter what happens to us, people understand. If you have a stroke and you start dribbling some of your food, would you want us to shut you away somewhere, or is that unfair? It is basic human values.

JG: How do the Green Houses support the Eden Alternative care culture?

AP: In culture change, we tend to deemphasize the physical structure of the building because too many people are building nice buildings and thinking they have succeeded in changing the culture when they have not. Organizations that build Green Houses come from all stages of culture change awareness. St. John's was the largest Eden Alternative nursing home in the world for ten years before they opened Green Houses. They had the culture in place even in their existing, old fashioned, hospital-like structure. The Green House environment served to support that culture. Others get excited about the Green House and begin building, but do not understand the culture that the structure was designed to support.

To quote my friend in England, a bulldozer is not a culture change tool. Having said that, the physical environment does matter, it does make a difference, it does cue people in good or bad ways. When you walk into a Green House home, you just relax. You do not feel like you are going into a hospital. Even as a clinician, you do not feel like you are going in there to do traditional doctor work. You just feel like you are making a house call. It gives you a whole different feeling and it is a very powerful, different feeling for the people who live there. The residents do not feel they are in a hospital ward. They feel as though they are living in a home, not a long-term care facility.

JG: What are your thoughts about the potential support ratio?

AP: I was researching the global aging demographic data and the potential support ratio changed my whole paradigm.

The potential support ratio, for my purposes, is approximately the number of working adults as compared to the number of retired adults. Who is earning an income and who is not? Who is living on a pension? The ratio is striking: from a ratio of twelve to one in 1950, it dropped to nine to one in 2000. By 2050, with the aging of the baby boomer generation, the ratio is projected to be four to one. It made it clear to me that we cannot continue to move older people to any kind of segregated community such as assisted living, nursing homes, or dementia villages. It is impossible mathematically because there will not be enough people to build, staff, and maintain all the communities. There will still also be a need for police, firefighters, doctors, teachers, and every other profession. The only solution to global aging is to keep people living with dementia in communities by creating inclusive communities.

The only solution to skilled care is to integrate skilled care and congregate living into larger communities so we can tap into social capital, because we will not have the necessary financial capital. St. John's is moving in that direction now. We need social capital. We need to keep communities inclusive. We need to keep people engaged so that most of them are contributing. The contributions do not have to be directly financial. People can volunteer, mentor, babysit. There are many solutions such as time banking. We need to focus on supporting those types of communities rather than building more assisted living and retirement homes.

JG: The retirement communities appear to be expanding rapidly.

AP: That is a dead end, and the problem is that aging will overwhelm us if we do not start building different systems. It is an issue that no one is addressing. That is why I keep talking about it in my publications and presentations. Another aspect of the support ratio is how to capture the knowledge, wisdom, and ability of the community that is dependent on some sort of care. Otherwise, we are creating excess disability among older people by marginalizing them. Support has to go beyond family ties for the system restructure to be sustainable. We are a mobile population these days, and families often live far away. An inclusive system will have to include neighbors looking after neighbors. My mother is almost ninety. She lives in the house I was raised in, which is about ten miles from me now. I visit her when I can. My daughter works at her house often and gives some personal assistance. It is great that one of her neighbors will run to the store for her if she needs something. The neighbors have a key and can check on her. Another neighbor will come over and do yard work for her or simple repairs when I am away. To me that is a healthy system. We need to start helping each other out more that way.

JG: Do you think it is important to create intergenerational connections?

AP: Yes. St. John's Meadows is the independent living campus and is about a mile from the home. Several years ago, Nazareth College began teaching a sociology course called Aging in Society in one of the common rooms at the retirement community. The residents who are interested attend the course. While the students and professors are talking about aging, they have the real aging experts in the room. Nazareth College won a national education award for this synergistic program. We hear more and more about moving older people to college campuses and moving students over to senior living and trying to blend those opportunities. They are wonderful ideas.

JG: Where do you give presentations?

AP: I present all over the world at conferences and seminars. I also teach a two-day course based on my books that is generally offered through the Eden Alternative. I have taught that course in seven countries. I've also taught it in Kentucky, Tennessee, Mississippi, South Carolina, Georgia, Texas, Illinois, and Oklahoma. I have received several Centers for Medicare and Medicaid Services grants to teach the courses in the US. Presently, I am consulting with Schlegel Villages in Canada. They are committed to person directed living. They have residences around Ontario ranging from Toronto to Windsor. I provide ongoing consulting support with dementia education and culture change.

JG: Are the communities at Schlegel Villages designed to look like villages?

AP: Yes, they have interior streets, many types of gathering places, and neighborhood areas. They are devoted to culture change for their employees and residents. They are for profit and are very mission based. I attended a marketing celebration dinner that they had in the spring and they were giving out awards for occupancy. The village that won the highest occupancy award for 2015 had maintained an average annual occupancy of more than ninety-nine percent. There were several others that were in the ninety-eight and ninety-nine range. They are highly respected.

JG: Please discuss the two-day dementia course that you offer.

AP: I wrote the original course five years ago and have recently revised it, with the help of Sonya Barsness, Karen Stobbe, Denise Hyde, and Laura Beck. It was based on my first book. I have expanded it to encompass a lot of the concepts in the second book as well. The course is two days, resulting in fourteen and a half contact hours. It is an intense course. Ideally it is great for twenty-five to forty people, but with the national grants, we have had classes of two hundred. Eden educators in the room act as co-facilitators and we break the tables into neighborhoods so we can work in semi-large groups. We have ten modules over the two days, beginning with relationship and team building. We explore the different views of well-being from the point of view of the resident. We talk a lot about dementia and challenge the standard way of caring for those living with dementia. I share some basic medical information, but very little, because that is easily available elsewhere. I challenge the narrow biomedical view and introduce my experiential view. We begin talking about paradigm shifts and basic culture change.

Then day two really jumps in with detailed information about face to face techniques, including communicating and facilitating tasks with people. Then we explore other ways to understand distress. What does it really mean when people say they want to go home? What does it mean when people are removing their clothes? What does it mean when people appear to be hallucinating or delusional? Those actions are all a form of communication or expression. Then we have a well-being exercise where a participant explains a real life challenge they are experiencing in their residence. I break the class up into the Eden Alternative Seven Well-being Domains and we determine which aspects of well-being are not being met. Then the participants work to design a plan that only proactively provides each of those domains of well-being, without specifically trying to address the distress at all. This enables providers a way around the blind spots that exist when one is focused on the behavior rather than the cause of the behavior. When behavior is considered communication, we look at it differently and we respond differently.

JG: Thank you for this interesting discussion.

AP: Thank you.

— END OF INTERVIEW —

Dementia Village

An interview with **Eloy van Hal**

Background

As part of a series of case studies on best practices in elder care, Sofia Widén, program manager of ACCESS Health Sweden, visited De Hogeweyk, the dementia village in Weesp, the Netherlands. De Hogeweyk was established in 2008 (Phase 1) and 2009 (Phase 2). The village provides high quality elder care services for individuals diagnosed with advanced or severe stage dementia. De Hogeweyk is the only dementia village in the Netherlands. The village in Weesp houses one hundred fifty-two residents in twenty-three small houses.

At De Hogeweyk, the care philosophy begins with small groups of individuals. Six people reside in each house. Living together in small groups enhances the quality of life for dementia residents. The residents choose the type of lifestyle they prefer. This may be an urban lifestyle or a traditional lifestyle. Each house combines individuals who have adopted similar lifestyles. A common lifestyle creates a social bond through a sense of familiarity and peace. Every house is equipped with a kitchen, a living room, a hallway, bathrooms, and individual bedrooms. Residents share the living room, the kitchen, and the bathrooms. Each house also has a shared outside area. Individuals can move freely inside and outside their houses. The residents can also walk around freely inside the village. Besides different outdoor streets, parks, and squares, the village includes a hairdresser, a supermarket, a café, a restaurant, a bar, and a theater. De Hogeweyk strives to create a typical community atmosphere. A guard prevents the residents from leaving the village.

The care philosophy at De Hogeweyk focuses on normalcy and autonomy. The caregivers support individuals mostly in determining their own rhythm. Some individuals prefer to wake up early. Others prefer to wake up late. The residents have breakfast at different times, although lunches and dinners are served according to the rhythm of the day, the preferences of the group, and the lifestyle choices. The caregivers cook and maintain the lifestyle in each house. Each caregiver tends to work in only one house. This structure helps the caregivers develop a strong relationship with the residents.

De Hogeweyk places little emphasis on curing dementia and treating its symptoms. Instead, its care philosophy focuses on residents' wellness and lifestyle. The residents can join various activities in the village, such as drawing or music appreciation. The majority of the residents are members of at least one activity. Individuals pay extra fees to enroll in additional activities. It is a combination of living, well-being, and care. The village has professional caregivers and practitioners to support the teams and residents in every house, but they also encourage and invite residents to be as active as possible with social contacts and normal household activities.

The dementia village obtains reimbursement from the Dutch insurance providers. The cost of living at De Hogeweyk equals the cost of other care homes for individuals who suffer from dementia. The average cost per resident in the village is six thousand euros per month. Private donations and sponsor funding helped establish the dementia village.

The founders of De Hogeweyk transformed a traditional nursing home into a village with a focus on quality of life rather than medical treatment. The founders realized that dementia is a chronic illness, which means that wellness and lifestyle are just as important as medical interventions. All employees wear normal clothing rather than uniforms to enhance the sense of normalcy in the village. Employees support the residents and do not exert authority over them.

Primarily, De Hogeweyk is a nursing home that adheres to all the standards of care established by the Dutch government. The dementia village upholds all nursing and rehabilitation standards, as well as other specifications within the care regulations. For example, the village employs a full time general practitioner who is specialized in geriatric medicine. A physiotherapist assists with keeping everyone mobile. The psychologist and social approach coach work closely together and advise on lifestyle matters and behavioral aspects of dementia.

De Hogeweyk differs from a traditional nursing home because De Hogeweyk gives the residents a sense of normalcy through the design of the village, the small scale houses, and its care philosophy. Thus the appearance is not that of a nursing home but of a normal village. The average length of stay at De Hogeweyk is about three years. There are thirty-eight to forty new residents who come to De Hogeweyk each year. Many volunteers come from outside the city of Weesp to participate in life at the village and to spend time with its residents.

De Hogeweyk has several entertainment venues, such as a theater that outside companies can rent for various events. Interaction with towns surrounding Weesp supports the atmosphere of normal life. At times, there are many people in the village. Other times, the village is quiet. The restaurant inside the village is open to the public for lunch and dinner.

The following interview with Eloy van Hal, previous facility manager at De Hogeweyk, senior managing consultant, and founder of De Hogeweyk, describes life in the dementia village and its care philosophy. This interview describes the concept of care at De Hogeweyk and the layout of the village.

About Eloy van Hal

Eloy van Hal worked in the dementia village for more than thirteen years. Mr. van Hal started as the facility manager at De Hogeweyk in 2002. At that time, De Hogeweyk was a regular nursing home. Mr. van Hal worked with the other founders to develop the initial concept and the layout of the village. As the facility manager, Mr. van Hal was responsible for the living and well-being of the residents of the nursing home. He and a care manager oversaw the daily operations of De Hogeweyk. Since July 1,

2015, Mr. van Hal has worked as a consultant at the Vivium Care Group. The dementia village is now a part of the Vivium Care Group. Due to growing interest in the care philosophy of the village, Mr. van Hal guides many visits to the village, gives talks at conferences, and also assists other care organizations around the world that want to adopt parts of the care philosophy of De Hogeweyk. Before joining De Hogeweyk, Mr. van Hal worked in another Dutch nursing home for about five years. Prior to that, he was the assistant manager of a cleaning company in Volendam for two years. Mr. van Hal studied household and consumer sciences at the University of Wageningen and facility management at Academy South in the southern part of Holland.

INTERVIEW

Sofia Widén (SW): Could you tell us a bit about your background?

Eloy van Hal (EVH): I completed my studies in household and consumer sciences at the University of Wageningen and also studied facility management at Academy South in the southern part of Holland. I was an assistant manager for a cleaning company and worked at another Dutch nursing home before starting De Hogeweyk. I started De Hogeweyk and the dementia village in 2002 with some colleagues. I was initially the facility manager for the village and specifically studied the surrounding environment of the nursing home. Since 2015, I have worked as a consultant at the Vivium Care Group. I have always been interested in elder care improvements.

SW: How do you measure the outcomes, results, and improvements in the quality of life at the dementia village?

EVH: Outcomes and results are an interesting discussion. Our point of departure from the standard way of measuring is to use common sense. We observed that working as a traditional nursing home did not improve the residents' quality of life. So my colleagues and I asked ourselves several questions: How would we like to live? Would we rather live in a larger group or smaller group? Would we like to eat home cooked meals or outside food? Would we like to have a daily routine?

My colleagues and I started our new model with a focus on lifestyle. We all agreed it was important that the residents could walk outside and make their own choices. Almost all of the methods we used to provide care were later proven to produce better outcomes than traditional care models. For example, six years ago we found published research that showed people eat better in smaller groups of about six people. We had considered a similar approach twenty years earlier.

Daily life challenges individuals who suffer from severe dementia. A traditional nursing home environment or hospital is confusing and stressful. The world seems dangerous. We made people more comfortable by making their world recognizable and safer. Research later supported our idea that smaller groups and a normal routine help individuals by creating a comfortable, familiar environment.

Exercise also has a positive impact on an individual's quality of life. We encouraged residents to walk around the village every day. We also prioritized social contact with others. Here in the village, residents walk around, meet each other, and talk with visitors from the outside. Research later proved that exercise and social interaction improve the quality of life. All these aspects are part of our philosophy.

There has been no research project that has proven the entire concept of De Hogeweyk model. However, individual components of our care philosophy are proven to produce satisfaction, to reduce anxiety, and to positively improve quality of life. I encourage you to walk around the village and see what is going on here. I want you to observe the individuals in the village. This way, you will understand better what I mean. Research and proof are important. Politicians normally change policies based on evidence. We continue to work to produce evidence in support of our care philosophy.

However, intuition and common sense are important, as well. I urge people not to wait until research endorses a care concept. Start with common sense. Ask questions and think about what you would like to have as you age. Many people from around the world show interest in the care concept at De Hogeweyk. I think that shows that we are developing something worthwhile. We cannot guarantee success in all areas of the De Hogeweyk care concept. However, we can examine individual aspects and measure their outcomes.

SW: In Sweden, the names of everyone diagnosed with dementia are entered in a registry. Doctors and nurses record a patient's symptoms, behaviors, psychology, and diagnosis in the registry. This system offers a standardized method of keeping records and providing treatments according to a patient's individual needs. Do you have such quality registries in the dementia village?

EVH: We do register the symptoms in our patient records. Such records enable caregivers to focus on aspects of care for each individual. However, such registries start with the idea that everyone is the same and needs the same type of care. After that, caregivers experiment with different interventions based on the registry records. The care model at De Hogeweyk acknowledges that everyone has different habits and different preferences for music, food, and daily rhythm. A common care system can adjust very little to accommodate an individual. The concept of the dementia village is to try to understand each individual and find out what makes them happy.

SW: Can other countries use the dementia village model?

EVH: Currently, a lot of western European countries think

in medical terms. These countries focus more on the traditional, medical, nursing home system. The quality registries
are part of this model. The dementia village represents a shift
toward holistic care. Risk prevention uses indirect methods
rather than direct medical intervention. However, other
places around the world gradually begin discussions focused
on quality of life.

Other countries can look at the De Hogeweyk model. The
dementia village should inspire others. However, they should
not copy our model exactly. Other countries should consider
the background, setting, and context of their own care society. People should work to understand the basic six pillars of
the De Hogeweyk philosophy and see how those elements
would fit in their country. Countries should not simply try
to replicate the entire design and care concept of the village.

SW: What would you like to improve in the village?

EVH: Some individuals suffer under the constant stimulation of people and movement. Residents that suffer from
frontal lobe syndrome are less likely to experience less agitation and stress in the dementia village. Even a small group
of five people might create too much stimulation for some
individuals. In our experience, they are sometimes better off
in a single room without much stimulation. They may need
to have walls painted white, a simple table, and a chair in the
room. De Hogeweyk is a social relational model, rather than
a medical model. A model with social and natural sensory
stimuli. For most of the people these are positive stimuli.
For some people with frontal lobe syndrome, they are not.

Living in a small group with a natural, recognizable daily
rhythm helps residents to cope with and structure their daily
lives. This keeps them away from boredom and loneliness.

Most human beings are socializers. But for some residents
who are not interested in socializing or are unable to live in

a small group, the dementia village is not ideal. Such individuals should live in their own small apartment in the safety of the village with all the freedom, facilities, and support. We have plans to build these types of rooms in the village in the future. These apartments would include a living space with a bathroom and a kitchenette. Residents would rent the apartments and arrange for care just as when they lived with their families. The Dutch insurance system would reimburse the residents or their family for the care. Insurance would also provide services that cater to individuals who want to live independently.

The independent residents could also request that De Hogeweyk arrange care but still benefit from a more individualized care approach. For some people, this type of individual living leads to loneliness. However, others prefer to live independently. Some residents spend more time in their own bedrooms than with other residents. For residents who like to do things on their own, an individual apartment might be the ideal arrangement. Future individual apartment designs might also include some social elements for residents who want interaction, but still want a separate living space.

Another improvement might be an even more open connection with the larger society. We are working a lot with schools, and have opened a restaurant, a polling station during election time, and much more in De Hogeweyk for the local community. We can improve, for instance, by building a day care center for children, or even a school. I think changes such as these would improve the village.

[Eloy van Hal shows Sofia Widén around the village.]

We are standing in front of the main street. As you can see, there is a shop, a hairdresser, and other normal amenities. Residents live their own lives in De Hogeweyk. They wander or walk freely around the whole village. Everybody who is working in the village, volunteers and employees, are responsible for the residents. We all look after the residents while they are walking and wandering around. We all keep an eye on them. We support them when needed. We also invite the residents to normal daily activities such as going to the supermarket for groceries. The village model makes it possible to socialize, to meet other people on the street or in club life. Sometimes residents even visit other houses. Sometimes they stay over for dinner. The caregivers in each house communicate with each other. After dinner, caregivers help residents find their way back home. The dementia village concept allows people to make their own choices and to meet other people with similar interests and hobbies.

Residents, together with their families or relatives, decide which activities to join. Some activities are available on a walk in basis. Most of the activities (such as classical music, painting, swimming, or baking) include approximately ten people. Some activities (such as film club, bingo, or going for concerts in the theater) have around fifty people in the group. The dementia village offers thirty-five different activities. The event officer for each activity arranges everything and collaborates with the caregivers and volunteers. The volunteers make sure that residents show up for the activities and help keep track of time if residents need that assistance. The caregiver will ensure that residents do not forget which activities they joined and schedule another appointment at the same time. We also have volunteers to assist the club leaders during the different activities.

SW: Could you tell me more about the volunteers?

EVH: Volunteers come to the dementia village to help De Hogeweyk and its residents, and to be a part of the village. The volunteers can help in different areas. We have six specific profiles for volunteers: club life, event office, maintenance, bus driver, church, and support at home. Some volunteers are here most days of the week. Others work twice a week either mornings or evenings in a house. Some help with cooking breakfast and lunches. Some work in club life and support the club leaders with activities. The dementia village becomes part of the volunteers' social lives. De Hogeweyk has around one hundred and forty volunteers.

Volunteers are a key resource. With more volunteers, De Hogeweyk can provide more service, more choices in club life, and better logistical support.

SW: What role does the family play?

EVH: The families play an important role. At De Hogeweyk, the family can become a normal family again. They do not have to be the caregiver anymore. The families are more than invited to act and behave as a family, to pick up the old rhythm of visiting mom or dad, making coffee, helping with the daily activities, or going out somewhere.

SW: What activities are offered here?

EVH: The dementia village has around thirty-five different clubs, including a painting club, a swimming club, a walking club, a bakery club, an outdoor club, a going to the market club, a film club, and a classical musical society. Other clubs include the café club, a high society club, a reading club, a cooking club, and a church club, among others. Individuals also choose from activities such as dancing and movement, music and songs, bingo, or day trips. According to the Dutch care regulations, the care organization must provide thirty minutes of activities per week. At the dementia village, hobbies and activities improve quality of life. Social events matter for many people.

Residency at the village includes the cost of one club. Residents may pay for additional activities. These additional payments only cover the costs of the activity. For example, a resident would pay twenty-five euros for swimming club as an additional activity because that covers the cost of the bus they ride to the swimming facility. A club leader, one of the staff, supervises each club. Many colleagues in the Netherlands questioned the benefits of many different clubs. They mistakenly believed that the residents would not pay for club memberships. Most individuals in the village pay for additional activities as an important part of their lives.

SW: How do residents spend their money?

EVH: This is a lengthy discussion. A resident's spending habits depend on each individual's family. Some families spend more than others. Families receive a monthly invoice for the costs of the activities. The invoice amounts range from zero to two hundred forty euros per month. An average invoice is seventy-five euros per client. Five percent of our residents spend two hundred forty euros every month.

SW: Are most residents members of a club?

EVH: Eighty percent of the residents are members of one or several clubs, which is about seven hundred memberships. Membership allows residents to join planned activities and walk-in events.

I would like to show you where the classical music group meets for their weekly event. Here residents can listen to classical music or watch the classical music performances on television. We decorated the room specifically for the classical music group, using antique chairs, elegant curtains, and carpets. We believe that residents can better absorb the classical music if the décor of the room creates an appropriate atmosphere.

SW: Yes, I can see that people would enjoy listening to classical music here.

EVH: The décor of the room encourages people to stay and listen during music appreciation time. All senses matter in care. Two weeks ago, I walked by this room. I saw a group of ten people listening intently to classical music. They looked happy. This is what they want, a quality moment. The swimming club strives for the same experience. Swimming is about doing something active instead of sitting in a chair.

Now, I would like to show you the restaurant. This restaurant is another important aspect of the village. The restaurant connects the residents to the outside world. The people visiting the village can also eat here. In the future, I would like to make the restaurant more visible to attract more individuals from outside the village to eat here more frequently. I have many ideas for improvement. If you come back in five years, I hope to have implemented some of these new ideas.

SW: What would you like people to know about De Hogeweyk?

EVH: When people come here, they only see the bricks and the stones of the village. They see the design. The dementia village is not only about the bricks and the stones. It is also about the care of individuals. I believe De Hogeweyk gained recognition because of its changes to the care approach and to the design of the care home.

We have a few core values that we refer to as pillars of care: favorable surroundings, lifestyles, life pleasures, health, volunteers and employees, and organization. The organization must work as a whole to implement changes. The management team must have the courage to challenge the existing rules and push boundaries within the laws and regulations.

When I go around and talk about the care concept of De Hogeweyk, I first explain the concept of care and talk about our findings. I tell people not to copy our concept straight away. I suggest that they adapt our concept to their own society, learn about our care pillars, and focus on quality of life instead of medical care. We encourage others to improve our concept and design, to improve our thinking. If other organizations skip the medical model, they can focus on the individual model. Look at the lifestyle choices of people rather than at the illnesses alone. Use common sense when looking for ways to improve the quality of life for people with dementia.

SW: What changes and opportunities in elder care do you see for the future?

EVH: The focus on risk presents a major challenge. Many policies focus on mitigating risks in elder care. Until policymakers find a solution and a cure for dementia, they will focus on safe surroundings. A guarded community is safe. We have built a village with normal surroundings and a neighborhood. We want the dementia village to resemble the normal world, but the normal world is not one hundred percent safe.

Perhaps we can use technology to improve safety in the future. For example, someday it may be possible for a taxi driver to recognize an individual who suffers from severe dementia. Perhaps he will see this information on his phone and take extra care while a person with dementia is crossing the road.

We need to work together with the community to raise awareness about dementia. Everyone should be aware of the symptoms. Once we raise awareness, we can discuss risks and risk prevention. This would enable the people with dementia to have greater personal choice and express preference, thus improving their overall quality of life. We can build an open, dementia friendly community. We want to create an integrated village where people who do not suffer from dementia can rent an apartment. We can have a mix of individuals. In the same way we create a safe environment for children, we should create a safe environment for individuals suffering from dementia. Decades into the future, I imagine we may not even need dementia villages. Perhaps we can just create dementia friendly communities. That is a vision for the future.

SW: Thank you, Mr. van Hal, for sharing your thoughts with me. I have had a great time in the dementia village.

EVH: You are welcome back any time. Thank you for listening.

— END OF INTERVIEW —

Dementia and Farm Life

An interview with **Gerke de Boer** and **Annie Herder**

Background

This interview is part of a greater research effort into dementia and best practices in elder care in Northern Europe. Sofia Widén traveled to the north of the Netherlands to study the innovative thinking at Cornelia Hoeve, a farm that is now a care home. In this interview, Gerke de Boer and Annie Herder explain how people with dementia live in Cornelia Hoeve.

Cornelia Hoeve is an old farm house which is now home to about twelve people with dementia. The philosophy of Cornelia Hoeve is centered on the well-being, personal freedom, and unique qualities of each person. The care vision of Cornelia Hoeve focuses on the living environment. Cornelia Hoeve is designed to improve well-being. The residents can walk in the garden, help with daily household chores, and continue their normal routines. The residents can decide at which time they want to wake up and if they would like to eat together with other residents or alone in their room. People working at Cornelia Hoeve establish close relationships with the residents. In this interview, Gerke de Boer and Annie Herder describe their approach. Mr. de Boer foresees that robots will be used to a much greater extent in the future in daily living and in care settings.

About Gerke de Boer

Gerke de Boer has been caring for elderly people in the Netherlands since 1971. He now runs a business that trains nurses in caring for people with dementia. Mr. de Boer trains the nurses that work at Cornelia Hoeve.

About Annie Herder

Annie Herder was the manager of Cornelia Hoeve from 2012 to 2016. She now works at a care home called Hof en Hiem. Her specialty is the care of individuals with dementia. Mrs. Herder has worked in elder care for many years; in 1970, she began in the first Dutch nursing home designed for people with dementia in Nieuw Toutenburg. She worked in different hospitals, nursing homes, and a children's rehabilitation center thereafter, and attained higher degrees in both Nursing and Management along the way.

INTERVIEW

Gerke de Boer (GB): My name is Gerke de Boer. In 1971, forty-five years ago, I started caring for the mentally disabled as a male nurse. After that I worked for four years in a large psychiatric institution. Then I worked four years with children. In 1982, I started working for the nursing home in Noordbergum, the Netherlands. At first I thought I would only do this for two years. It smells a little in those homes and it was boring. I stayed there for sixteen years. Within half a year I was completely sold on it. I have now had my own company for four or five years.

Sofia Widén (SW): What is the name of your company?

GB: My company is Gerke de Boer Bij- en nascholing. We train and coach nurses working in dementia care. Another group which is growing very, very fast in the Netherlands is psycho-geriatric individuals. That group is going to cause an enormous number of problems over the next ten years.

210

SW: Are there care organizations that can provide enough support for psychiatric care?

GB: There are some organizations. In 1958 the government started to not let people live in big institutions in the Netherlands. Instead, people have stayed at home for the last twenty five-years. They are growing older now. I interviewed ninety of these mentally ill individuals throughout the Netherlands, from the south to the north. I also wanted to capture cultural differences. What we saw was that these people need to go to nursing homes because they cannot deal with the complexity of society anymore.

The first three people that I interviewed, I thought I was in a movie. I asked the first person why he had come to live in a nursing home? He said because UPC—that is a broadcast company—changed the channels so that the NetherlandOne television station was not on button one anymore. The television is their only connection to society. They sit in their flats and call up UPC. However, they are answered by a robot giving them a menu. In twenty seconds the voice on the telephone gives them four more options. It makes those people crazy. When you are very fragile, and many are in a very bad mental condition, that literally makes you crazy, especially when you already have a lot of problems like falling asleep.

SW: That is why the first people had to move in. What about the second and the third?

GB: The first person I interviewed told me about UPC and I was not surprised. I am a psychiatric nurse and I have heard those stories a hundred thousand times before. The television is watching me. Complete paranoia. Then the second person also said UPC changed. That's when I thought, "Where is the camera?" Then the third said the same to me and that was the first time that I thought it might be true.

SW: So you think the reasons people move into care homes can be strange or absurd?

GB: It's not just dementia. The ninety individuals I talked to symbolize a far bigger group of elder people who will be coming into the nursing homes over the next ten years.

Most of the time the people come because they start forgetting to take care of themselves. They do not shower anymore. They do not take their pills anymore. They do not eat anymore. They do not brush their teeth anymore.

Annie Herder (AH): They do not take care of themselves.

GB: They do nothing at all. That is the reason they come to nursing homes. They cannot take care of themselves.

AH: My history is the same as Gerke's. I also worked in Nieuw Toutenburg, but that was long ago. For the last seven years I have worked for Care Center Hof en Hiem. Hof en Hiem consists of four residential care facilities and three small scale residential facilities.

Cornelia Hoeve is one of these small scale residential facilities. This care home was a farm. The number of residents who suffer from dementia is growing at all four residential care facilities. Cornelia Hoeve opened in September 2012. During the month before that, the building was renovated. This farm grew very fast. We try to keep it as residential as possible.

SW: Do they eat breakfast here and lunch in the kitchen?

AH: Sometimes. They like to sit here to have a full view of the garden. The ceiling is glass. There is plenty of outside light. It brightens the indoor areas. People who suffer from dementia like a lot of light. This is why a glass ceiling was installed.

Our vision of dementia care is focused on the living environment. Scents, colors, shapes, lights, and sounds have a major effect on how people feel and behave. The brain of dementia sufferers is particularly sensitive to this. We cannot do anything about the condition, but we can control the environmental factors. That is our vision. The more pleasant the environment, the less demented the behavior. The furniture, the lights, the garden—it all looks pleasant. The residents can walk a lot. In the front part of the house is a kitchen and a living room. In the former stables there are twelve apartments.

SW: Why is colored furniture used here? Is it to create a contrast?

AH: The contrast, yes. When people have dementia, their sight gets worse so they cannot see all colors. But red, for example, is a color you can see for a long time. Dr. Anneke van der Plaats, a famous geriatric doctor, said to me that you need to look through the eyes of the person with dementia. Then you see how the individual is looking at the world.

SW: Has she written books?

AH: Yes. Gerke and Anneke also wrote a book together, *The Demented Brain*.

SW: Why is there a TV in the middle of a darker room?

AH: The idea of the movie house is Anneke van der Plaats's. The intention is that residents can continue their own life as much as possible by providing them with a home-like, family environment with emphasis on providing assistance in every-day life focusing on the needs of the residents. The residents' well-being is key in this respect. We can make sure the residents can live here in the most pleasant way possible so they can still enjoy the last years of their lives. They can stay here until the end.

SW: Is the farm for everyone or is it mostly for individuals who are used to living out of town?

AH: It is for everyone with dementia. It can be different, but some people who have lived their life in Amsterdam come here and they want to live here.

SW: Do they retire here?

AH: Yes.

SW: Has anyone ever moved to the farm and said, "This is not for me."

AH: Once, in the beginning.

SW: Why was that?

AH: He was very aggressive. He needed more room, more space.

SW: Might some people feel more secure in a smaller environment?

AH: Each person has their own apartment, but they are not often here. They are always looking for each other in the living room.

GB: They like to go out and see the other residents and interact with them and be together.

AH: Activities also include cleaning the house, doing the dishes, and doing the laundry.

SW: Do they like to work in the garden?

AH: Yes. Next to the farm there are gardens where you can work. Other activities are organized as well. Residents live a sheltered life here. They cannot leave because the door is locked. It is safe. I like the small scale. Many of the people I think are happy.

GB: There is no fixed structure.

AH: We follow the rhythm of the residents. If they want to sleep until seven, it is ok. If they want to sleep until eleven, it is also ok. When they want to have a meal in their room, it is ok. When they want to have their meal with other people, it is ok.

SW: Do you believe that larger care homes can be as flexible as you are?

AH: That is a good question. It is very easy to say, "The kitchen closes at eleven," but it is really a question of, "Do I work where you live, or do you live where I work?" Regular nursing homes tend to become institutions. I think care homes can achieve more than you might think.

GB: When you want to change a system, you do not need to discuss the things you want to put into the system. You just need to talk about the things you do not want to do anymore. One of the main things we should stop in those homes is medicalizing care. It is a problem of the highest order that cure and care are fixed together. The cure is poisoning the care.

There is a difference between a good life and a healthy life. Every helper, every nurse, every doctor in these institutions thinks that a good life is a healthy life and the other way around. If people live a healthy life, they will have a good life. I think the success story here is that there is more attention to the relationship between the nurse and the resident. That is what is happening here.

SW: Would you say you should focus not on the illness but on the person?

GB: Yes, and on the relationship with the helpers. That is the secret here. The helpers here, the nurses here, they feel confident letting people sleep until nine or ten. They know it is ok. These organizations also care for the nurses. This is one of the secrets of good dementia care.

SW: How do you create trust?

GB: Just do it. Tell them we work this way here. We will help you take good care of these people. We select personnel to work here who are focused on dementia care, which is very different from other kinds of care.

SW: What is your latest project?

GB: We are now working with elder psychiatric individuals. Not people with dementia—psychiatric individuals; people with severe anxiety, depression, psychosis, and fear. It is very, very new. There are no books in the Netherlands about how to work with this group.

SW: Are you optimistic or pessimistic?

GB: I am very optimistic, especially about the use of robots.

SW: Why robots?

GB: Robots improve life, especially for elder psychiatric individuals. Within five, six, seven years, every person here will have a personal robot. That is going to be fantastic.

SW: How will robots help?

GB: In every way.

SW: Reminders?

GB: Yes including reminders. The robot will need to recognize if a person is sad, glad, happy, or worried. A brain that is damaged like a dementia brain can be misled easily. When they see a robot smiling, they really think it is a smiling person. That is why elderly people with a doll think it is a real baby. There used to be a person here who had a little seal with a battery. That guy walked around with this seal for three years. It was alive for him.

AH: Robots help with taking medicine, doing exercise, keeping people alert.

GB: Yes. So I am very optimistic about that.

SW: A final question. What would you like to improve?

GB: This is ideal. This is one of the top locations in the Netherlands. It is small, it is cozy, and it has very good nurses. There is a sound vision. There is a clear direction. It is modern. It is open. I think this should be the standard in the Netherlands. I do not think we could do any better. You will never make everybody happy.

SW: Thank you so much for your time.

GB: Thank you for visiting.

— END OF INTERVIEW —

Improving Dementia Care and Care of the Elderly

An interview with **Linda Martinson**

Background

Aleris is a private health and social care company and one of the largest providers in Scandinavia. Aleris manages three hundred and fifty health and social care centers in Sweden, Norway, and Denmark. The company employs about ten thousand people. Aleris operates in specialist care, primary care, diagnostics, elder care, and social care, with an annual turnover of seven and a half billion Swedish kronor (about nine hundred and forty million US dollars).

Since 2010, Aleris has been owned by the Swedish investment company Investor AB. The aim of Investor is to develop Aleris so that the company continues to deliver sustainable, high quality care. In 2013, Aleris and Investor created a foundation to promote research in patient centered care. In the future, the company hopes that research can discover new methods to improve and sustain high quality care.

Aleris elder care offers care homes, homecare services, and home healthcare. Aleris elder care focuses on patient capabilities, preferences, needs, and values, not on illness. The company aims to provide care that is respectful of and responsive to individual patient preferences, needs, and values. The focus on patient centered care ensures that patient values guide all clinical decisions at Aleris.

The Swedish municipalities use tax money to fund Aleris homecare services, home healthcare providers, and care homes. The municipalities distribute the tax money between private and public health and social care providers according to the Freedom of Choice Act. The act gives Swedish citizens the right to choose between private and public homecare and home healthcare providers. The chosen provider receives reimbursement from the municipality.

In this interview with Linda Martinson, manager of an Aleris elder care home in Stockholm, Sweden, she talks about quality registries, national guidelines, and the development of new and better methods in elder care. Ms. Martinson discusses how to treat patients suffering from dementia with respect and dignity.

About Linda Martinson

Linda Martinson works at Aleris as the manager of Odinslund elder care home in Stockholm. She holds a degree in nursing from Mälardalen University College. Prior to her nursing studies, she obtained a master's degree in Germanic languages from Stockholm University and worked as a professional translator. In 2008, Ms. Martinson began to work as a nurse in elder care. After two years in nursing, she began her current work as a manager of elder care homes.

INTERVIEW

Sofia Widén (SW): Thank you for your time. What is a usual work day like for you?

Linda Martinson (LM): I start my day with a walk around Odinslund. We have six units at the elder care home. I talk to the staff to get a sense of what the day will be like. I ask the staff if there were any problems during the night, if any relatives have been here, if there have been any complaints, or if something good happened. Every day is different in elder care. We take care of people with dementia. Their conditions change from day to day. It is important to get a sense of what your workday will be like at the beginning of the day. I also talk with relatives.

An important part of our work is to understand the development of dementia and what kinds of symptoms the elderly can have. For the rest of the day, I do normal administrative work and attend weekly meetings. We also arrange social activities for our nursing homes, such as parties, singing groups, and painting circles. These activities help raise the quality of life for the people who live here.

SW: How many people work here, and what kind of care home is it?

LM: Odinslund is an elder care home with a total of forty-six residents. We employ fifty people. We have staff on duty around the clock. The major staff group consists of nurses, head nurses, assistant nurses, and physical therapists. Odinslund operates one nursing home and one dementia care home. We have sixteen residents with physical limitations in the nursing home. The dementia care home has thirty apartments.

Our patients with dementia have their own apartments with a bathroom and a small kitchen. The apartments create the feeling of living at home.

At Odinslund, we also have activity rooms where the patients can eat together and watch television. Three assistant nurses are responsible for the daily activities. The assistant nurses work with activities that stimulate and provide social meaning for the patients. The assistant nurses have different profiles. One nurse specializes in physical activities, while another one specializes in food. We also offer gymnastics and nature walks.

SW: How do you work with food at the dementia care home?

LM: We work with food in different aspects. It is important to look at the environment. It is important to have a calm and peaceful environment when we serve food to patients with dementia. When there are too many people eating at the same time, these patients start to focus on the environment instead of the food in front of them. It is important to work on these different dimensions.

Studies also show that classical music stimulates appetite. We listen to classical music when we eat to create a peaceful atmosphere that surrounds you. We also use different colors. People who suffer from dementia appreciate the contrasts on their plate. Potatoes, meat, and salad are nice colors together. The different colors of the food help our patients to understand what they are eating. One symptom of dementia is that you are unable to remember information. It is important to be concrete and distinct in the way you serve and present the food.

SW: Do you use the quality registries at Odinslund?

LM: Yes. We use one quality register to estimate weight, malnutrition, risk of fall, and risk of developing bedsores. We use another quality register to record the behavior symptoms of dementia patients. We also use a palliative care register that measures how we handled the process before dying and how we integrated the relatives. We then learn if we listened to the last wishes of a dying person. That is important for us to learn from. In Sweden, we use registries for research in our daily work at the nursing homes to record data and to standardize care.

SW: What happens to the data that you record in the quality registries?

LM: I can see the quality registries for my unit. For example, once or twice a year, we record the number of people in my unit who fell. We can see if it is the same person falling and what we can do to prevent this person from falling again.

In palliative care, it is important that we learn from our mistakes. We must learn how to reduce and prevent symptoms. We try to integrate everyone into our work, so that we learn from each other. Assistant nurses work closely with the patients in their daily life. These nurses must be able to analyze and understand the symptoms. Twice a year, we compare the results of the quality registries for the unit on a national and municipal level. It is an inspiration for us to see that we achieved better results than the average municipality.

SW: Do you also know how long it took to heal bedsores or what kind of treatment you used?

LM: Yes. In addition to the quality registries, we record information in patient journals. We can then return to the journals and check for relevant data. Recording statistics is important for us. It is also important to incorporate the right skills in our care homes. For example, I recruited a nurse specialized in bedsores. Her competence helped us to reduce and heal more bedsores. Quality registries help us to receive a regular baseline.

SW: Five years ago, did you use quality registries in Sweden?

LM: Yes. Quality registries were introduced in Sweden about five or six years ago.

SW: Do you know if the homecare staff at Aleris also uses quality registries?

LM: I do not know, but the quality registries are available.

SW: Are healthcare providers required by law to use quality registries?

LM: No. Healthcare providers follow the national guidelines of the National Board of Health and Welfare. The goal of these guidelines is to contribute toward patients and clients receiving a high standard of medical care and social services. Swedish healthcare providers take for granted that everyone follows these guidelines.

SW: We talked about environment, food, and music. How would you improve the national guidelines for these areas?

LM: I would change the restrictions related to food preparation at elder care homes. The national guidelines restrict us from handling raw proteins. Instead, we must order prepared meat for the elderly. The smell and sound of cooking makes people feel better. If we could prepare food for the elderly at Odinslund, our patients would feel more at home.

I would also change the restriction against walking outside alone. Elderly people that move to a care home feel deprived of their freedom. At Odinslund, we try to open up as much as possible, but we restrict our patients from leaving the building alone. People who suffer from dementia can be a danger to themselves. It is important to supervise and secure the environment. At Aleris, we try to improve our elder care homes with gardens. Spending time in the garden, the elderly stimulate both body and mind. They can pick berries or exercise at an outdoor gym. Even patients over ninety years old benefit from exercise. Exercise improves patients' balance, which prevents them from falling.

SW: Do you take patients out for a walk?

LM: Yes. We organize daily walks. We also provide group walks, twice a week. It is important to remember that the elderly are in different shape. Some people are unable to join the walks. We try to find other solutions for them. Physical activities and outdoor activities are some of the most important life quality parameters for the elderly. The National Board of Health and Welfare also recommends physical activity in the national guidelines.

SW: How do you organize care for the thirty residents who live at your dementia care home?

LM: At Aleris, we match dementia patients with a contact nurse. The contact nurse stays in contact with the patient throughout his or her life. The nurse also stays in contact with the patient's relatives. The contact nurse is like a lawyer for the patient. On the first day at the dementia care home, the contact nurse writes an implementation plan together with the patient's relatives. The plan covers the rights and interests of the patient. The plan also outlines the patient's routines. All employees have access to this implementation plan.

It is important to secure continuity among the staff. Each unit group consists of five employees. We never rotate our shifts. Instead, we make sure that the same group of people works with the same elderly patients. Each unit group knows the routines of their patients. The group knows the expressions and the symptoms of the elderly with dementia.

The patients in our dementia care home exhibit many different kinds of behaviors. Some dementia patients are aggressive, while others are worried or anxious. Some of these patients walk around and greet people, while others sit down and keep silent. There is a lack of research in patient centered care. In 2013, Aleris set up a foundation to promote research in this area. In the future, I believe we will establish units specialized in meeting the needs of patients with particular types of behaviors.

SW: How do you equip assistant nurses who arrive inexperienced? How do you make sure they know how to handle all these different symptoms and people?

LM: Qualified nurses have an important role in our elder care home. They are the highest medical advisors available. Once a week, a consultant doctor visits our elder care home to advise the nurses. We always recruit nurses with experience. We require work experience of one to three years in emergency care, elder care, or orthopedic care.

It is also important that we think of our patients as palliative care patients. Elder care homes do not have the goal of healing our patients. Instead, we create quality of life. Our patients have multiple diseases, or else they would not be here. We must create a safe environment where we can ease the patients' symptoms.

It is important that our nurses understand their role. At Aleris, we offer regular competence training for our nurses. Three times a year, all nurses attend training in palliative care and ulcer care, for example. We have both in-house and external trainings. Aleris also provides network meetings for the nurses. During these meetings, nurses from different units gather and discuss recent dilemmas.

SW: Do you work with the Queen Silvia Foundation?

LM: Yes. We have contact with them. We took part in a dementia conference arranged by the foundation. The conference discussed the importance of knowledge and how to work in concrete ways with dementia patients. The foundation inspires all sorts of palliative approaches to dementia care in Sweden.

SW: How do you organize care for the sixteen residents at the nursing home?

LM: These residents have a physical handicap when they arrive. Some even develop dementia while they live here. This is a different type of patient, one who can express what he wants and what he needs. The staff at the nursing home works differently from the staff at the dementia care home. The nursing home staff needs to listen actively to the patient and then give him the support that he needs. At the nursing home, we also see depression and fear of death among the patients. Depending on the patient's life circumstances, the assistant nurse or contact nurse can sometimes take the patient to church.

SW: Do you offer any kind of conversational support to help with depression?

LM: Yes. Conversational support is a task for the assistant nurses. Our doctor sometimes also gets help from a psychologist. We do not have a psychologist on staff, but sometimes we hire them as consultants.

SW: Is depression or social isolation a problem at elder care homes?

LM: Yes. We can see this problem in the yearly national report on public health called Open Comparisons. The report compares indicators related to living conditions, living habits, and health effects on the municipal and county council levels in Sweden. Open Comparisons gathers patient satisfaction information through a questionnaire. We then receive the results from the questionnaire for our residents. Open Comparisons is a good tool for us to learn how to work with our patients.

This year, the results showed that our residents are satisfied with my staff. The results indicated that my staff is empathetic and follows the needs of the patients. Our patients still suffer from isolation and struggle to find meaning in life. This is a hard task for my staff to address. Imagine arriving at an elder care home with seven other unknown patients. The other patients may not be the people you would choose as your friends. Then you have staff coming from other countries, with other cultural competencies. You may experience cultural clashes for the first time.

In the future, it will be important to find a meaningful environment. Patients arrive at the elder care home with an empathetic, nice, and competent staff that starts to take care of them. Soon, the same patients will have no functional autonomy in life. No one needs them. Everybody takes care of everything for them. That makes them stop seeing the meaning in their lives. They feel like a burden on society.

This area needs to develop. If patients can keep their autonomy, they can keep their freedom. At Aleris, we work with assigning small responsibilities to each patient. One person is responsible for handing out books, while another is responsible for making the table. These people then feel that they are needed. Even small everyday tasks matter. To be needed is a central human desire. It makes you feel good.

SW: You mentioned the development of methods in elder care. Can you explain this development for someone who is unfamiliar?

LM: In Sweden, we use many elder care methods. We developed a method called Bekräftande förhållningssätt, inspired by the validation therapy method. The basic principle of the method is the concept of validation or the shared communication of respect. For example, when you meet a person with dementia, he or she can ask if you would like to start an ice cream shop together. The obvious answer would be "No. You are too old and living at an elder care home." However, instead of stating the obvious, answer, "Yes I do," and continue to support his or her ideas. You then enter the reality of a person with dementia. This makes the person feel peaceful and respected, without feeling corrected. The individual's integrity is preserved, even if she lives in her own reality. Last year, we tried that method and it worked well.

SW: How can you measure the effect of this validation method?

LM: We measure the behavioral and psychological symptoms of dementia and how much medication the patient needs. One common medication is sleeping pills. If we enter the imaginary world and live the dream or desire of the dementia patient, we meet the person in his or her reality. By doing this, you can reduce their symptoms of dementia, reduce their medication, and improve their sleep.

The problem is that people suffering from dementia are unable to channel their feelings. The feelings of restlessness and anxiety may be an expression of feelings of worthlessness or confusion. It is important to create an environment for these people where they can feel safe and comfortable.

SW: Who developed the validation therapy method?

LM: Naomi Feil developed the validation therapy method in the late 1960s. She is still alive and lives in America. Her method is mainly directed toward people in palliative care or people with severe dementia. In Sweden, this method inspired us to develop our own methods tailored for people with dementia. These methods are successful social innovations.

SW: What other kinds of methods like this do you use?

LM: There are many methods that we can use. Reminiscence therapy is one example. It is a method of recalling past experiences to support dignity. All people in elder care can work with these social innovations. We try to look at the whole person and to meet the needs of her soul. The reminiscence therapy helps our staff to go deep into the history of a patient to see what she achieved. For example, if a patient worked in music, the staff can set up a collection of musical instruments. The patient can then play her favorite music and try to pick up old memories. This can also be inspiring for a person who has not talked about music for a long time.

SW: Have you also tried to introduce information technology into your dementia care home?

LM: Yes. We plan to be part of a research project, together with

Ersta Sköndal University College in Stockholm and a company called eLOTS. eLOTS is a small company that develops applications (apps) to educate elderly people on their tablets. The aim of the app is to train people with dementia to remember their daily routines. For example, it can be a lesson in how to use the toothbrush, how to use a razor blade, or how to put on your socks in the morning. We want to develop an app where you can see these lessons on a tablet every morning. Then we want to analyze how this affects patients' ability to perform these routines during the day.

SW: That is very interesting. When do you plan to start this project?

LM: We hope to start in February 2016.

SW: You mentioned the lack of research in the field of patient centered care. Do you feel that you have to push the development of elder care on your own?

LM: Yes. That is also what makes it exciting. There are many possibilities to improve the quality of elder care and attract more people to the market. Today, elder care is a low status work area in Sweden.

SW: Is there anything else you would like to add to this interview?

LM: As a manager, we focus on relatives with their complaints and on society with their media coverage. I believe it is equally important to listen to your staff. Managers invest large amounts of money on equipment, education, and staff. However, you must have high employee satisfaction to deliver a high quality of care. Staff members daily affect your budget results when they care for people, make medical judgments, and support relatives. It is complex and hard work to run the daily operations of an elder care home. Managers must support and inspire their staff to continue working. I think managers must rethink the way external factors affect us and instead start to focus on our employees.

SW: Thank you very much, Linda.

LM: Thank you.

— END OF INTERVIEW —

Elder Care Technology

An interview with **Bo Iversen**

Background

As part of a series of case studies on excellence in dementia care, Sofia Widén visited Denmark to study Danish companies and organizations. This study is part of a larger research effort in dementia care in Northern Europe.

In this interview, Bo Iversen, Sales Manager at Life-Partners, discusses the new software and planning tool, IntelligentLIFE, which Life-Partners recently introduced. IntelligentLIFE was developed jointly by ANYgroup and Life-Partners. Life-Partners previously developed a software system called Life Managers. ANYgroup is a producer of smart sensor technology. These companies work together to provide services to the Rise Care Home, a technologically advanced elder care home in the south of Denmark.

In 2013, the mayor of Aabenraa City, Tove Larsen, invited Life-Partners to provide an innovative solution for the care home. The innovation that Bo Iversen presents in this interview focuses on communication with relatives, the needs of the user, and the care planning structure used by professional care workers. By using big data and algorithms, the IntelligentLIFE design can prevent falls, set passive and active alarms, and help care providers develop non-medicinal interventions instead of relying on medications. This type of software can also help reduce loneliness since it provides a means for users to connect with family members and friends. This service is a way for relatives and staff members to structure care routines, and for individuals to engage in more diverse activities.

About Bo Iversen

Bo Iversen is a partner at Life-Partners. Mr. Iversen is also the Sales and Marketing Manager at IntelligentLIFE. Prior to this, Mr. Iversen worked as Sales and Export Manager at B&C Textiler Aktiebolag. Earlier, he founded and served as the Chief Operating Officer at Cost:bart. Mr. Iversen also owned the largest sports store in Aabenraa, Denmark, SportMaster.

INTERVIEW

Sofia Widén (SW): Please describe IntelligentLIFE.

Bo Iversen (BI): IntelligentLIFE is a new product developed by two Danish companies: Life-Partners, which I represent, and a company called ANYgroup. ANYgroup specializes in sensor technology.

SW: How does the system function?

BI: Intelligent sensor technology can generate alarms and detect early risks. Life-Partners created a communication and planning design around intelligent sensors for people and their relatives, for caregivers, or for the municipality.

SW: Who buys the design, the person who lives at home or the care home?

BI: Both. We started in nursing homes. Now we are also serving those who live at home. People like staying in their own homes, plus the municipalities do not have space for all their elderly. We found a way to help people stay longer in their own homes.

SW: How long have you worked with the municipality?

BI: Three years now. We have nine employees.

SW: Who founded Life-Partners?

BI: My partner, Lars Jessen. Life-Partners was founded in 2009. The company was looking into the health and fitness world, making communications systems between fitness centers and their members. When Aabenraa built Rise Care Home, our mayor at that time, Tove Larsen, asked if there were companies in the area who could help the municipality. Lars, my colleague, contacted her. The mayor asked about improving communication within the nursing home and with the relatives outside the nursing home. That is how the collaboration began.

SW: Did you have prior relevant experience?

BI: We had a little experience in fitness, but not in elder care. In a fitness club you have employees and you have members. Then we added relatives.

SW: Please describe your services.

BI: We place the person in need of care at the center of the design. That is very important. A lot of other solutions say they do, but they do not. Other companies develop planning tools for staff. It is important for us to put the people who live in the home at the center. The important thing for people in need of care are their social and professional relationships. We have combined these relationships into one solution to offer higher life quality and safety to the resident. This applies to falls and other dangerous situations, but it also means simply feeling safe. Security means everything.

The intelligent sensors are installed in different places in the home or nursing home. A person can just push a button and say, "I need help." Once the alarm goes off, caregivers come and help the user. You can set the alarm to alert relatives or municipal officials or caregivers. You can send alerts first to relatives and then to the caregivers if you prefer.

We also have bed and wall sensors. Some elderly people are not comfortable leaving their beds when their lights are off. The sensors detect you leaving your bed. We can put the light on in the hall or in the bathroom immediately. When you return to bed, we turn off the light.

We have a kitchen sensor for the stove. We can detect the difference between smoke and steam. We have a heat sensor. If the heat sensor gets too warm, we can turn off the stove remotely. The technology is smart. It knows if a person is at home cooking or if someone has left their stove turned on.

SW: What is the origin of the sensor technology?

BI: The sensor technology relies on algorithms. If you are sitting up in bed, we can detect this. If you are not in one of two places, sitting or lying down, then we know you are not in bed anymore. The sensor only registers movement. We have a software algorithm with all the data that comes from the sensors. This helps us detect falls early. The algorithm generates the alarms.

A person can leave his or her bed without triggering an alert. If that person is not back again within ten minutes or fifteen minutes, we will send an alert to the nursing staff or to relatives. We can also send the alert immediately when you leave bed; but if you leave bed and we detect you in the bathroom then we can start the timer again. It is all customizable. The sensor itself is not intelligent. The algorithm behind the sensor is intelligent. That is also how we use it for early detection. We help prevent falls. If you leave your building at night, we can send an alert.

If you are not in the kitchen at all during the day, you might become dehydrated, you might not eat or drink. We can send a warning to staff or to relatives. If we have a sensor in the room, we do not see if you are moving over here or over there, but we can see that you are moving. For early detection, maybe for sleep, that is the best way to see how you are doing. The algorithm learns your sleeping pattern.

SW: Does the algorithm recognize deviations from routine?

BI: Exactly. The sensor can tell us if you sleep well, given your normal sleep pattern. We can see if you are starting to become sick, if you are anxious. If your behaviors deviate thirty percent from what is normal for you, then we send an alert. We can use the design as a dialogue tool. We understand what is happening in your life. Maybe you typically go to the bathroom once a night. Now you do it four times a night. Are you getting an infection? Is something wrong?

Once the system has been in your house for twenty-four hours we have data. After we have been there for two weeks we have more data. We can personalize a care routine for you. Our doctoral student analyzes our system to produce a quantitative study. We can change medicines or care based on your needs and your data. Any devices with a ZigBee specification can be plugged in, such as a blood measurement device or a wearable device. ZigBee is a way of making two things talk together. We can use other formats as well, but ZigBee is very standard. I think there are about two thousand compatible products now.

There is no person who looks in on your behavior. No one sees what is happening in your daily life. The software only follows it. You can tell us that you would like us to alert someone if your behavior changes by thirty percent.

SW: Do you have user feedback?

BI: Yes. We receive a lot of feedback on the use of our platform. Users are very happy with it, especially the alerts. The system develops better care routines. One lady was in pain every day. The care workers had stopped listening to her. Our system discovered that she was in pain because she never slept more than forty minutes at a time. We alerted the care workers, who brought in the doctor. The doctor administered new medication and the lady started sleeping again.

The important thing for us is the algorithm and the application that handles all the communication and care planning. The advantage is that IntelligentLIFE is not only an alert system. It is not only an early detection system. It is a communication planning system. It is a social medium. It is a holistic solution.

SW: Please describe the social element in more detail.

BI: You need to manage all your appointments. You also need to order food through whatever system as well as with the municipality. That is a lot to handle for an elderly person. You as a relative like to help your mom or dad, but it can be very difficult because of the distance. You call them and you take them to appointments.

We give them a program with a single login. Then they have the whole plan in one place. They can start with the app. Now we can plan. We can communicate with the municipality. We can communicate with the relatives. The person has a way to see the relatives—a daughter or son, family nearby, even the neighbors. This also includes friends, old colleagues, and volunteers. There are a lot of organizations that want to help. It is very difficult to get them in contact with elderly people who are starting to have issues leaving the house. Once they start having symptoms of dementia they do not leave the house much. All kinds of relatives want to help the person in need of care. They just do not know how to help or how to plan. Maybe you as a daughter want to visit your father this week. With our system, you can see that the neighbor is coming on Monday and another friend is coming on

Tuesday. Then you know that it might be better if you came on Wednesday or Thursday.

SW: Is coordination important?

BI: Yes. Coordination is very important. If you are not living with your father, you become anxious. Is he falling? Is he getting up in the morning? How is he doing? It might be good for you if he receives a small sensor package so you can know if he has fallen. You would receive an alert. Is he going outside at night? You would like to know.

Living with a person with dementia can be very hard. Now they cannot tie their own shoes anymore. The relative living with the person in need of care is taking on new care jobs all the time. It can be very stressful. We install the system for them and they can let the person with dementia stay at home alone. They can turn on the system and go away for social events, activities, and other things and come home fresh to help take care of the person with dementia again. If they fall or leave the house, we alert the neighbor or caregivers or whoever. That really helps the family.

SW: Does your system work for a person who has mild dementia, or is it designed specifically for people with severe illness?

BI: I think you need to see it in two ways. The earlier you start using the app, the better the elderly learn to use it themselves. I think the most important people to learn it are the caregivers and the relatives. Sometimes the people with dementia do not use the system. Sometimes they can use it and other times they cannot. Maybe they can use it with the caregiver or with the relative.

We have people with dementia who are using it. It will be much easier for younger people because they use technology and apps all the time. My dad is sixty-seven. When he stopped working two years ago the first thing we went out to buy together was a smart phone and a tablet phone. Now he uses them all the time. We have started talking about whether he should give the system a try so that we can know what is happening in his life. Should we help him learn now, while he still does everything himself? When should we start using it? We want to be able to help, especially when he is living one and a half hours away from us. It is important that we know what is happening in his life. Not to monitor him, just to help him and support him.

If you go through the system briefly you can see how intuitive it is. The contact people all have different colors. Pink represents caregivers. Blue stands for relatives. Yellow will be other people. When you select one of them, you can write a message or send a video request so you can talk about the issue at hand.

SW: Can you chat and talk using your system?

BI: Yes. With solutions like this, when you are using video and communication, you gain a certain level of security. More than just the person and the relatives use these things. The municipality and the caregivers are also involved. Your security increases a lot. It is easy to understand what is written. It is easy to create new messages. You just choose whom you want to send messages to from your contacts. Then you write your message. You can speak and receive your messages from a tablet or a smart phone as well.

SW: Can you dictate messages?

BI: Absolutely. Then we have the pin board. This is sometimes called the elderly Facebook. In many homes in Denmark we have homecare. When caregivers are in the home or in an apartment in a nursing home there is a book in which the employees can write to relatives. For example, the person may need shampoo or something else, whatever happened that day. But you need to be in the room to read it as a relative. We have created this pin board. It is like Facebook. You write a message and when you post it all the people can comment on it, like a thread. This is instant communication with all of this person's contacts at one time. All his contacts go in and see what is happening on the pin board. He can write on it himself. Relatives and employees can write together. Some use it mnemonically, as a shopping list. We have some elderly who are really into it. They write ten posts a day. This allows the family to follow what is happening. It also gives them better contact with their grandchildren because they are much more mobile.

SW: Can one user connect with another user? Can an individual who lives at Rise Care Home add another individual who lives at Rise Care Home?

BI: Yes. Another thing that is really popular at the care homes is the menu. They can check the breakfast, lunch, and dinner menus. They post what they are going to eat for lunch, for instance. They take pictures of it. So if it is carrots, there is a picture of carrots with meat and potatoes. I know one woman who does this very well. Every morning she goes in and she says, "What is for lunch today?" They also include a description of the food.

If you are going to take your dad for a visit, or you go out into the city on a trip, you can go into the system and say, "I am unsubscribing my dad for lunch on Saturday." Now you do not need to call the nursing home and say, "On Saturday you do not need to make lunch for my dad." You'll see that the box is unchecked and you receive a confirmation message that he is not expected for lunch. Also, as a relative you can buy your own meal for the day or coffee or something else. You can say, "I will come and eat with my dad." You can come eat and buy your own stuff. There is also a personal gallery where users can have their training program or family pictures.

SW: Could your father who lives at home call his nurse or his doctor through the system?

BI: Not his doctor. The municipality buys the system, and the municipality only employs nurses. If they are in the system, you can communicate with them.

SW: Might a general practitioner buy your system and log in?

BI: Yes. There are two parts to our business strategy. One is to sell our system for use in municipalities and small private care facilities. Our second strategy is to sell the system to consumers directly. Individuals as well as care systems would like to be able to monitor and assess their people remotely. Our system also allows individuals who live far away from their parents to involve neighbors in the care.

We are using the system on my street. An elderly woman recently became a widow. Her two sons live a two-hour drive away. She has Parkinson's disease and also a little dementia. She has friends in the neighborhood. We are all connected to the system. We use the system to see how she is doing. Her sons can track her progression and decide when and if she might need more help. Eventually we hope our municipality will purchase the system so that she will have access to nursing and homecare when needed.

SW: Do you think hospitals and general practitioners will be connected in this way in the future?

BI: I think that is in the future. Maybe the person will use our system and the hospital or the general practitioners will use another more suited to their needs. Then we will need to coordinate communication. That may be a solution. I have a friend who is a doctor. He says, "I am paid for everything I do. If I need to go to the nurses and do it another way, then I do it in two different systems. It takes longer. In the end, I receive more money for it." The technology is not integrated.

240

SW: Would doctors need to be paid to answer an email or take a phone call?

BI: Yes. We have initiated a program for family welfare to allow the system to assist a family caring for a sick child, for example. The mom and dad will be contacted by many different professionals. Physiotherapists or nurses want to make appointments with the family. The family needs to arrange all the visits. They could use help.

SW: Will they use the system as a planner?

BI: Yes, as a planner. Twenty different people want to contact the family. They have just learned that their child is sick. The family is grieving. Now they need to handle all this. In these three months, you are not only meeting with someone one time, but many times. Then you need to learn how to take medicine, when the nurses are coming, and everything else. The system can help the family plan everything.

SW: Do you deliver services abroad?

BI: Yes. In Germany and in Norway. We have our own development strategy. We have customers in Denmark, Germany, Norway, and Greenland. In March we won an innovation prize in Germany called Altenpflege. It is the biggest fair for elder care in Europe.

SW: Thank you for your time.

— END OF INTERVIEW —

Rise Care Home

A case study based on interviews with

Kirsten Springborg and Mette Pawlik Olesen

Introduction

As part of a series of case studies on excellence in dementia care, ACCESS Health visited Denmark to study Danish companies and organizations. This study is part of a larger research effort on dementia care in Northern Europe.

Rise Care Home (Rise Parken) strives to be at the forefront of dementia care. The home consists of eight houses, with twelve people in each house. Eighty percent of the residents at Rise Care Home live with dementia. Residents who suffer from extreme symptoms of dementia, such as aggression, and those who face challenges being part of larger groups live in separate houses in order to ensure the right environment for them. This separate house is split into two smaller units containing a maximum of six residents each.

About Kirsten Springborg

Kirsten Springborg works as coordinator for welfare technologies in Aabenraa Municipality. She has served in this position for over five years. Prior to this, Mrs. Springborg worked as project coordinator in Aabenraa Municipality for six years. Before she worked in this position, Mrs. Springborg was a district leader in the same municipality.

About Mette Pawlik Olesen

Mette Pawlik Olesen works as a Change and Process Consultant. Her core expertise centers on strategic communication, crisis communication, and change communication. She has worked with the municipality of Aabenraa for about two years. Prior to this, Ms. Pawlik Olesen worked as Communications Coordinator at Sygehus Sønderjylland, the hospital in Sønderjylland.

TOUCH AND PLAY

The Touch and Play software program is large scale technology designed for residents of the Rise Care Home. Touch and Play was developed to support cognitive training for the elderly and people with dementia. The residents can walk up to the large dashboard and initiate an application at will. Residents can play games, watch movies, listen to songs, and access a range of other applications. Touch and Play was developed in close partnership with the private sector. This is one way Rise Care Home provides stimulation to residents through sound, music, and movement.

GYM, EXERCISE, AND PHYSICAL STRENGTH

Rise Care Home includes a gym for its residents. Residents may work with physiotherapists and a general practitioner to maintain physical strength and to reduce certain symptoms of dementia. The home has applied for money from TrygFonden to develop a new exercise program. Residents can sign up for the program, receive help with exercises, and develop their strength. The general practitioner measures the outcome, such as increased body strength and balance. In the gym is a motivation tree where each resident can hang his or her nametag once they have completed an exercise routine. Each unit at Rise Care Home competes every month for a prize, which is given to the unit that exercises the most. The gym is also available to staff.

LIVING AND ROBOTIC ANIMALS

Rise Care Home believes that animals can have a calming effect on individuals. For this reason, the home keeps guinea pigs and hamsters in the care home. Residents help feed and take care of the animals. The animals live in the middle of one corridor. The care home has also invested in PARO. PARO is a robotic seal that interacts with whoever is holding it. A stressed person can become more tranquil by interacting with PARO. Residents are only encouraged to interact with PARO together with a trained employee. Rise Care Home also has a robotic cat.

While Rise Care Home believes in a comprehensive technology strategy, that technology is always used together with employees. Technology is used as an integrated part of daily care and is never a substitute for personal care or warm hands.

WELLNESS NORDIC ROCKING CHAIR

Rise Care Home also houses the Wellness Nordic Rocking Chair. Residents who lie in the chair relax, listen to music, and feel the rhythm of ocean waves. These stimulants help calm residents who experience anxiety or other symptoms of dementia. Care home professionals participate when individuals lie in the chair. A nurse is trained to deliver sensory stimulation. A staff member presses the individual's hands, arms, and legs while the individual lies in the chair. The chair is positioned with a view of the garden.

WINDOWS AND GARDENS

Rise Care Home is built with large windows that stretch from the ground to the ceiling, often two meters or wider in breadth. The rooms are large and spacious. The care home is surrounded by green areas, gardens, and grass. The doors in the home remain open. Individuals can stroll freely into the garden, but once an inhabitant exits the garden a GPS sensor alert system sends a message to the staff saying that someone is leaving the care home. In this way, dwellers can experience freedom while staff members maintain oversight.

SNOEZELEN ROOM

Rise Care Home has a relaxation and experience room called the Snoezelen Room. A Snoezelen Room is an environment in which individuals can experience different stimuli. In the Snoezelen Room at Rise Care Home, individuals can experience a range of activities such as sitting in a massage chair or putting their fingers into sand and shells. The residents may also choose to watch a movie with footage of beautiful scenery, observe lights of various colors, lie on mattresses, or put a knitted blanket over their body to pacify them. Even more exciting, residents can view colorful water fountains and listen to the sound of water. This experience room is another part of the Rise Care Home vision to stimulate all of one's senses and to reduce the negative symptoms of dementia.

WELLNESS ROOM

There is a wellness room at Rise Care Home with a bubble bath, hair dressing facilities, and other related services. Next to the wellness room is a spacious garden.

GARDEN

There is a newly planted apple orchard at Rise Care Home. The garden overlooks the surrounding fields. The garden contains a music area where individuals can play their own music with outdoor instruments. Individuals can lie under a large tree and look up. Participants can take a stroll in the garden and sit in their own outdoor seating area. At Rise Care Home, the indoor and the outdoor environments blend and complement each other.

By design, Rise Care Home contains small units with independent doors. Yet, since there are eighty-four residents in all, the care home can draw on certain benefits of larger scale operations. With support from the municipality, the staff work constantly to adopt new technology.

In short, Rise Care Home is a model for care homes in Denmark and abroad.

Aabenraa Municipality

An interview with **Jakob Kyndal**

Background

As part of a series of case studies on excellence in dementia care, ACCESS Health visited Denmark to study Danish companies and organizations. This study is part of a larger research effort in dementia care in Northern Europe.

The municipality of Aabenraa is located in the Region of Southern Denmark. Its largest town and the site of its municipal council is the coastal city of Aabenraa. The municipality covers a large section of the Danish border with Germany. From 1864 to 1920, the region was part of Prussia, in the Province of Schleswig-Holstein, and as such part of the German Empire until the end of World War I. As part of the Versailles conference of 1919, it was decided that a plebiscite should be held in Schleswig to determine the demarcation between Denmark and Germany. The results restored Danish rule over the region in 1920. This created a German minority in the region, and to this day a large part of this minority lives in the municipality of Aabenraa, which also houses the minority administration. During the interwar period, Aabenraa also hosted the German minority government.

With the Danish Municipal Reform of 2007, a new and larger municipality of Aabenraa was formed through a merger. Today, the municipality covers an area of 940 km², making it geographically the ninth largest in Denmark, and totals a population of approximately sixty thousand citizens. Current estimates show that the population is likely to remain stable in the coming ten to twenty years, though general demographic changes might cause a slight proportional increase in older people. As of today, the proportion of the above sixty-five age group in Aabenraa is slightly higher than the national average.

Municipal Responsibilities

The Danish healthcare system consists of three separate pillars: The regional sector, which is divided into five geographical units, is responsible for secondary and tertiary care. The municipalities, of which there are ninety-eight in Denmark, provide healthcare and a variety of social and elder care services. The third pillar consists of general practitioners, who are privately managed.

In general, the public sector in Denmark is highly decentralized. It is based on the principle that as much as possible should be dealt with on a local basis. In practice, this means that a large number of public responsibilities and activities are handled by the municipalities. The primary municipal responsibilities under the governing body of the city council include healthcare and social care services, employment stimulation, integration, industrial and economic development, environmental and technological services, cultural services and recreation, primary schooling, and day care. The healthcare and social care services include rehabilitation, homecare, and promotion of health, as well as care for the elderly and disabled, social psychiatry, and the running of nursing homes and specialized institutions. Besides providing primary care and healthcare, the municipality also finances twenty percent of regional healthcare services. In practice, this means that if a citizen of the municipality is hospitalized, the municipality covers twenty percent of the hospitalization costs. This also applies to the elderly. The incentive is then to keep citizens healthy and to inspire them to continue living active, healthy, and independent lives in Aabenraa.

Jakob Kyndal, the Director for Social Care and Healthcare in the municipality of Aabenraa, manages an organization of approximately one thousand seven hundred employees in three main departments: the care and elder care department, the health and prevention department, and the disabilities and psychiatric department. The local government works with one unified mindset to provide person centered care. The municipality currently faces a growing complexity of healthcare challenges, both structurally and demographically.

A growing proportion of the Danish population lives with chronic illnesses. In 2005, just under forty percent of the adult population were living with chronic diseases. Based on recent estimates, almost forty-five percent of the adult population will be living with chronic illnesses in 2020.

The municipal government of Aabenraa has taken a strategic approach to the demographic challenges related to aging. Firstly, the government wants to stimulate innovation in the welfare sector. They do this by cultivating a local innovation ecosystem and engaging in public-private innovation partnerships, where the municipality sponsors innovative solutions that are developed and tested in practice in the care sector. Assisted living technology producers create new technologies in conjunction with end users and professionals through a practice oriented approach, where the citizens are an integral part of the innovation process.

The municipality focuses on organizational development and a thorough person centered care approach. As part of this effort, Aabenraa has built a specialized rehabilitation center as well as an acute nursing unit that collaborates with the hospital emergency department to support individuals who need urgent care. The municipality is also expanding intermediate care levels and investing in areas of psychiatric care.

Assisted living technologies and digital solutions are integral in the municipality of Aabenraa. The municipality has a long tradition of engaging technology innovators from the private sector and strives to be agile and dynamic. By cultivating a variety of partnerships with the private sector, the municipality of Aabenraa helps aging individuals to live at home independently for as long as possible.

The retirement age in Denmark is currently sixty-seven. The government is discussing a proposal to raise this to sixty-eight. It is clear that the Danish healthcare system needs restructuring and reform.

In this interview, Jakob Kyndal describes coordination challenges within the structure of the Danish healthcare system.

About Jakob Kyndal

Jakob Kyndal, MSc in Political Science, has been the Director for Social Care and Healthcare in the municipality of Aabenraa for seven years. Mr. Kyndal previously worked as Healthcare Director in the municipality from 2007 to 2009. He also served as the Executive Director of the municipality of Rodekro between 2003 and 2006. Before joining municipal top management, Mr. Kyndal worked in the Danish Ministry of Defense where he held numerous positions, including a three-year position at the Danish contingent at NATO.

INTERVIEW

Jakob Kyndal (JK): Denmark has three levels of government: national, regional, and municipal. I think this system is similar to that of Sweden and many other European countries. That being said, the center of the world is local. It has a little bit to do with the influx of technology. We emphasize that we are on the border of Germany and Scandinavia so we are kind of in a gateway position both mentally and geographically. That is one of our growth strategies. We use healthcare technology to create local growth. Such are the tasks of municipalities.

There are five divisions in this department. The three main operating units are the care and elder care department, the health and prevention department, and the department for disabilities and psychiatric services. These three departments total approximately sixteen hundred employees. In addition to this, we also have a department for rehabilitation and referral as well as a department for management and organizational development. These two departments total approximately one hundred employees who take care of referrals and overall management, direction, and communication.

Most municipalities have general practice coordinators who support cooperation with hospitals. General practitioners are not hired by the municipality as they are in Norway, where they have paid municipal doctors twenty hours per week. Hopefully we will be there in a couple of years. That way you actually have a local healthcare system.

In Denmark we have three individual sectors. We have the regional level with responsibility for the hospitals. We have the private sector with the general practitioners. Lastly, we have the local level of the municipalities. We spend a lot of energy coordinating between these three sectors. In truth, the two public sectors engage. We try to engage the private sector by other means, but different regulations and incentives apply to the private sector. Still, the division of tasks is regulated and we have a cooperative relationship with them.

Sofia Widén (SW): Do the organizations all operate under one umbrella?

JK: No. In terms of strategy, our regions and municipalities face pretty much the same challenges. Demography is a big one. Then we have what I call the structural challenges emanating from the system. These are built-in management problems and economic challenges. We wrestle with declining budgets, rising demand, and the rising complexity of healthcare challenges. We are trying to tackle as much as we can on our own while engaging partners as well.

SW: Do you raise taxes independently in the municipality?

JK: Yes. Raising taxes is a vital part of financing our daily tasks. Seen in combination with the challenges mentioned before, the only solution is to have the citizens do more and more themselves. We pull in new resources from civil society and empower citizens to live healthy longer with less support from hospitals and municipalities. On the national level, the working age population shows no growth at all. Simultaneously, we also have an enormous increase in the elderly population. Who is going to earn the money to support those who need care? At the same time, the national government imposes strict national regulations regarding the overall headroom for raising taxes.

The working population is pretty much stable. Looking ahead, the proportion of eighty-plus-year-olds will see a steep increase, as will the proportion of sixty-five to seventy-nine-year-olds. Everything else being equal, those people will cost more money. This is the national picture. I believe it is pretty similar to what the Germans are looking at now and the Scandinavians as well. We wrestle with the same problems. The welfare state is being strained.

In relative terms, the proportion of working age people is declining while that of the aging population is rising. A significant number of people are unable to find a job, need better or different education, or have become temporarily ill or otherwise incapacitated. When we talk healthcare initiatives on a municipal level, what we want to do is to make sure that the next generation of young people will all receive an education. The correlation between education and health is convincing. It begins with the youth. If they go out and find a job as a nurse in the private sector, they can earn some money for the rest of us. As for those who have a job but cannot hold on to it, we try to support them as much as possible. We try to bring them back to work as quickly as we can.

We just did an analysis of young people with mental problems. The number of eighteen-to-twenty-five-year-olds with some kind of mental problem doubled four times between 2012 and 2015. We need to intervene before they become uneducated adults. With respect to the elderly living longer, you are not considered old today when you turn sixty-five. We are going to delay retirement perhaps by years. When you are sixty-five or seventy-five you are still a resource for the rest of us. That way we can support the most elderly people.

SW: What is the retirement age in Denmark?

JK: It is sixty-seven today. I think it will become sixty-eight with the new government. If you look at chronic disease predictions for 2020 on a national level, you see a near forty-five percent increase in the adult population with one or more chronic diseases. That is another area of concern. If you correlate that with our local numbers, mathematically it means that we will go from four thousand one hundred today to a staggering seven thousand eight hundred people in 2025 with one or more chronic diseases. We are trying to help early on with healthcare and prevention.

We have embarked on a strategic approach to managing the future. Many municipalities take a similar approach. We need to reinvent welfare and we need to do it together with those whom it will affect. Cocreation is the name of the game. We have embarked on a new mission statement that is going to focus all seventeen hundred employees in the department on the same task instead of everyone running in multiple directions. What we try to do is instill the various disciplines with the same mindset, a rehabilitating mindset focused on working together with individual citizens.

We take a practically oriented approach to assisted living technology and development. We do it as part of daily business. We do not do it in labs. We let industry do that. For instance, they can go to Odense municipality to work on robots. What we try to do is simple. We do the development together with citizens. We tell industry to come to us because here we can provide a natural, practical, person centered environment where they can work directly with those who are going to use their solutions. We develop solutions together.

We tailor our technologies to people's needs. That is the

approach that we have embraced. It is tailor made to the needs of person centered healthcare. This is how we develop new welfare and healthcare solutions. Working with one common mission statement focuses everyone on the same notion of what this is all about and how we go about achieving it. The mission statement guides us in running a complex business that is comprised of people with numerous professional backgrounds and runs on a very large number of different computer systems.

We have seventeen hundred employees with perhaps thirty, forty, or fifty different educational backgrounds. How do we make use of these differences? We bring in a number of practically oriented experts together with citizens to find new solutions. For them to be able to work together, we need to develop new competencies among the staff. In order to make the money benefit the individual citizen, we also need to change our way of managing our economy and our reimbursement system. It demands a value driven approach. We need to create value while addressing the citizens' needs. In order to do so, we are developing our way of working effect oriented systems underpinned by efficient management. That is what we call a three hundred sixty degree organizational approach. You have to change culture, competencies, and information technology.

We need cross functional competencies in the future. We have new people coming in from universities, colleges, and schools, then we have the bulk of the people we employ today. Those are two different groups. We need to ensure that the people who have been here ten or fifteen years are up to date on their specialties. At the same time, we need to empower them to be able to work together across boundaries with other disciplines. Regarding the new tasks that are imposed on us by the hospitals and national authorities, we need to adopt new specialties. We take a three-tiered approach to the development of competencies: basics, cross functions, and specialties.

As an example, in order to manage the pace of development in the healthcare sector, we need to create acute nursing units in the municipalities to work together with the hospitals both prior to as well as in post-hospitalization. This requires new special skills to support treatment and rehabilitation at home, but also a broadening of basic nursing and care skills. We need to think in terms of early intervention and early diagnosis. The philosophy is that we must succeed in early prevention and early diagnosis, or even a step prior to diagnosis, to prevent hospitalization when possible.

Municipalities have to play a greater role in the future. We need an intermediate step after the hospital, before we send citizens back to their own homes or to the nursing home. And we need specialized teams to support continued treatment or rehabilitation at home. Acute functions are one of the stepping stone elements here. They take in citizens from the hospitals prior to sending them back home. We have a specialized rehab center for these challenges. On the other hand, our early prevention personnel can send people to acute care or to the rehab center in order to avoid sending them to the hospital altogether.

SW: Does the money go to the municipality in those cases?

JK: The big discussion is how much money goes to the hospitals and how much money goes to the municipalities when we talk about new tasks and rising complexity. We do not receive enough money in the municipalities, which means we have to work innovatively to find new solutions and lower costs per intervention.

SW: Do you have national funding options?

JK: Yes. It is complicated to apply for money. If you have a change in the law or a shift in responsibility, money follows that new responsibility to some extent. For the most part the central government and the ministries work with their own funding mechanisms. They earmark a certain amount of money, as they recently did for extremely elderly and weak citizens. Then they attach some expectations to that earmark. "You need to spend this money on acute functions. You need to spend this money on developmental competencies." All welcome suggestions to a certain extent, because the ninety-eight municipalities have ninety-eight different priorities. At the same time, it is a vital part of local government to maintain the right and obligation to decide on local priorities, for instance with respect to spending money on young people and not on the elderly.

We are expanding acute care and nursing homes based on both national and local funding. It is the same with respect to dementia. We can apply to various funding sources. We have done so and we have received money. This is a European Union sponsored project. German Danish businesses, nursing homes, the municipality, and educational institutions are all engaged in developing new solutions for people with dementia. I believe we have a total budget of eighteen million Danish kroner [two and a half million US dollars] over three years for the project. Forty percent is sponsored by the participating organizations and the other sixty percent comes from the European Union.

SW: If they sponsor development for three to five years, do you take over the cost thereafter?

JK: That is the tricky part. All these temporary funding arrangements pose a problem if you do not receive continued funding or if you do not somehow make a project sustainable, which is often a challenge.

SW: Do the acute nursing projects save money for the regional hospitals?

JK: Yes, to the extent that we can prevent or shorten hospitalization. The acute nursing and specialized rehab centers are part of our daily business. The municipality permanently funds them. In the formative year or two we got external funding support. We managed to make that funding permanent. It saves us money too. We cofinance twenty percent of the total cost of our citizens' hospital care.

SW: Is that an incentive to keep them here?

JK: That is exactly how the municipal finances are presented. The national government is going to correct this mechanism so that those municipalities who do not prevent the weakest elderly from needing to be hospitalized will pay a significantly higher price. That will be the new system starting in 2018. It changes the incentives and focuses on the elderly.

SW: Do demographics affect you?

JK: Yes. Being a predominantly rural municipality, we have a higher proportion of older people here than in the big cities.

We are working on creating a network of partners. One of the challenges is that we would like companies to relocate, pay taxes, and create jobs here. The competition is tough. Companies have certain requirements.

Over the last ten years, we have seen an increase in the level of education in the municipal healthcare sector. We work on recruitment and retention. With the transfer of certain healthcare tasks to municipalities, we need to gear up. The change is more or less incremental, but it is definitely a trend. We have increased the number of training experts and therapists of various sorts by twenty to twenty-five percent. Nurses are a scarce resource, so we may compete with the hospitals for the best of them. At the same time we have traditional home nursing, which is still common in Denmark. However, the increasing complexity and new tasks in municipal nursing will make us more attractive to the newly educated.

SW: Will focusing on more specialized skills attract them?

JK: It sends a signal that we have more complex tasks. You can build a career both vertically and horizontally in the municipalities. You can even crisscross sectors because you are more in touch with the general practitioners. The general practitioners place a high emphasis on the fact that we need more nurses. Our nurses support the doctors in virtually everything. We may actually come into a kind of competition with the private sector. The flip side of that is making it more attractive to work in the municipalities. In terms of the number of requisite skills and the volume of citizens in need of care, the municipalities have more than the hospitals. There are a variety of possibilities.

We do not have the answer to how we can attract young people, but we are very much attuned to the challenge. We have seen an increase in the number of new nurses over the last ten years, but that is relatively speaking. Moreover, we have also seen an increase in employees with various types of master's degrees in healthcare. Most are in public health. We did not see that many ten years ago. It is a new trend.

When we look at the age of our current employees, we see another challenge. In ten years' time, a lot of these people will not be here anymore. So we are very much focused on bringing in a new, younger generation.

SW: Thank you for your time.

— END OF INTERVIEW —

A Neighborhood Model of Care

An interview with **Jos de Blok** and **Gertje van Roessel**

Background

This is a summary of an interview with Jos de Blok, founder and chief operating officer of Buurtzorg, and the transcript of an interview with Gertje van Roessel, a nurse coach and international coordinator at Buurtzorg. The interviews highlight the Buurtzorg philosophy and working methods in homecare management. Buurtzorg methods are being replicated worldwide.

Buurtzorg Nederland is a not for profit homecare provider with a reputation for delivering high quality and affordable elder care services. Buurtzorg means "neighborhood care" in Dutch. Buurtzorg is centered on neighborhood resources, including family members and neighbors.

Buurtzorg was founded in Almelo, the Netherlands, in 2007, by a small team of nurses. It has since grown rapidly. As of October 2015, eight thousand nurses, organized as seven hundred teams, care for sixty-five thousand patients. The organization is expanding into other countries, including Sweden, the United States, and Japan. Many other Dutch homecare organizations are adopting several aspects of the Buurtzorg care model.

Buurtzorg provides patient centered care. Buurtzorg focuses on the needs of patients and patients' resources and networks. Buurtzorg also relies on professional staff, especially nurses. Buurtzorg nurses work in teams of ten to twelve nurses. Nurse teams are self-governing. Each nurse is a manager. The lean model of the organization is one of the keys to its success. Overhead costs are around eight percent. In 2012, Buurtzorg ranked first among all homecare organizations in patient satisfaction in the national quality of care assessment. Buurtzorg was also named the best Dutch employer in 2011, 2012, 2014, and 2015 by Effectory, a company that collects, analyzes, and uses feedback from employees and customers in the Netherlands.

Buurtzorg generates surplus income, which is used to fund innovation and expansion. One of the core principles of the care model is to unlock a person's own abilities to care for him or herself. Care is considered a success when patients care for themselves and nurses are no longer needed.

About Jos de Blok

Jos de Blok is a trained nurse. He holds a degree in healthcare innovation and recently received a master's in business administration. Mr. de Blok has a long history in community nursing, both delivering care and in management positions. From 2000 to 2003, he played an important role in the National Association of District Nurses. He led a movement by community health nurses to take responsibility for their own professional development. Mr. de Blok worked to create a clear vision of the role of nurses in primary care.

In 2007, he established Buurtzorg, together with his team of four professional nurses. In 2011, Mr. de Blok was named the most influential healthcare leader in the Netherlands. That same year, Buurtzorg received its first award as the best employer in the Netherlands by Effectory. Mr. de Blok has transformed home-based healthcare in the Netherlands. Today, Buurtzorg has grown to nearly eight thousand nurses, with teams in the Netherlands, Sweden, Japan, and the United States.

The Buurtzorg Philosophy

In the words of Mr. de Blok, "the idea of neighborhood care is to mobi-lize existing resources to create ecological systems of self supporting environments. In these environments, professional care is the only care people need. The focus must be on sustaining these dynamic networks."

Mr. de Blok described the core values of Buurtzorg this way: "What we try to do is quite simple. What is important in healthcare? When people suffer from a handicap, impairment, disease, or other health-care problem, it should be easy to receive support." He continues, "We need competent doctors, nurses, and healthcare professionals. The initial idea of Buurtzorg was to focus on the quality of life and quality of health of people, and the cost per client. If you have some sort of norm for quality of life, then you can judge what is a reasonable cost per client."

Mr. de Blok explained, "Quality of life can be complicated. I try to make it easy. Quality of life is what gives people satisfaction and empowers people to take care of themselves. Quality of life comes when people have enough social contacts and people in their environ-ment. Buurtzorg helps people to achieve a high quality of life. We focus on interventions that empower people to take care of themselves. Self care leads to fewer hours of inpatient care. We work with educated people who create dynamic networks in their neighborhood."

Of his unique approach to his workforce, Mr. de Blok said, "We need to provide healthcare staff with enough freedom to do what they think helps people. We need to work together. The current problems in health-care are nothing that one person can solve independently. I try to involve everyone, including patients and nurses. If several people in one neigh-borhood struggle with the same problems, we may develop collective programs to support these people. I think we started an important pro-cess that led to an international discussion on how we are doing this."

According to Mr. de Blok, the important thing is to simplify the healthcare system. "Try to see the relationship between someone who needs something and someone who gives something. Healthcare hap-pens in this process. I recommend that you read the book *Reinventing*

Organizations, by Frederic Laloux. This book will help you to under-stand the simple healthcare process. Mr. Laloux writes from an orga-nizational perspective. He believes that the current way of organizing leads to a lot of problems. Society needs grassroots thinking. The focus should be on the operations. *Reinventing Organizations* describes how this practice developed into a higher level of consciousness, organizing with different membranes of self management. The book is a best seller and sold all over the world. *Reinventing Organizations* is one of the best books on this topic."

Mr. de Blok continued, "In my opinion, hospitals must shift their focus from service delivery to management. This shift in focus has proven successful in healthcare organizations that have adopted my philosophy. I met with six chief executive officers. It is important that the chief executive officers have been nurses because they under-stand what healthcare is about. They have support from their staff. Other chief executive officers lack this credibility. The solution is to simplify healthcare organizations. If you are creative and connect social problems, then you can provide healthcare."

Mr. de Blok explained the simplified organization of Buurtzorg: "We disconnected the financial part from the professional part. We do not get paid for everything we do. Instead, we created an organiza-tion where the revenue is enough to cover all necessary costs. We are structured differently compared to other healthcare organizations. Our organization is flat, with fewer levels of hierarchy and lower overhead costs. At Buurtzorg, the overhead costs are eight percent, compared to twenty-five or thirty percent at the average healthcare organization. We only have well-educated healthcare workers. Our staff members design their own care methods based on what they see in the community. Our staff members each have skills in different methods. As a result, we can spend more money on the education level of nurses. We can also spend more time on networks supported by internet and social media. We can provide healthcare to everyone, even to people without insurance or citizenship. We help people. Now many refugees are coming to the Netherlands and Europe. We will help them as well."

Mr. de Blok spoke about the big picture and his plans for Buurtzorg: "It is our responsibility to contribute to better healthcare. In the Netherlands, Buurtzorg reaches fifteen to twenty percent of the population. Soon, we will reach fifty percent. It is just a matter of time. We do not need to set targets. We expand to nearby villages, cities, and neighborhoods where Buurtzorg is present. We are continuously expanding in the Netherlands as well as abroad. We want to provide the best homecare support. Thank you for taking the time to understand our care."

About Gertje van Roessel

Gertje van Roessel is a nurse coach and international coordinator at Buurtzorg. After receiving her bachelor's degree in nursing from the University of Nijmegen in 1983, she began her career as a nurse for a psychiatric hospital in the Netherlands. Ms. van Roessel also completed two postgraduate degrees, the first in healthcare innovation and the second in healthcare management. She later worked as a community nurse in the northwest region of the Netherlands and as a care manager for different private organizations. Ms. van Roessel joined Buurtzorg in 2007.

INTERVIEW

Sofia Widén (SW): Tell me about your professional background.

Gertje van Roessel (GR): In the 1980s, I wanted to become a district nurse. A district nurse is a nurse with specialist training, while a community nurse works at a patient's home instead of at the hospital. It was difficult in those days. It is hard to imagine that today because of the shortage of district nurses in the Netherlands. Instead, I started work as a community nurse for about seven years. When I think back to my time as a community nurse of the 1980s, I realize that the district nurses at Buurtzorg work in a similar way today.

SW: In what ways do the district nurses at Buurtzorg work similarly to the community nurses in the 1980s?

GR: My work as a community nurse was simple. We had our autonomy. We worked in the small neighborhoods. We had our colleagues. The management team was located far away. The management team left us alone without a lot of rules and regulations. Instead, we arranged our work for ourselves. Families, doctors, everybody knew us in the village. We involved and maintained close contact with the whole neighborhood.

Afterward, I saw changes over the years. More organizations with community nurses merged and became bigger. The front-line people lost contact with the organization and struggled with the new administrative work. Nurses spent less time on what they were trained to do. We needed to think more carefully about the needs of patients. I saw increasing fragmentation of nurses' responsibilities. Early in my job, I saw assistant nurses replacing experienced nurses. The assistant nurses took care of intakes, assessments, and official partners. The experienced nurses did the planning. The nurses with more education spent less time with the clients. The management team thought the experienced and highly educated nurses were better at desk work and coordinating the assistant nurses. The less educated assistant nurses did all the work with the patients.

When assistant nurses were brought in to replace the experienced nurses, patients suffered. No one was responsible for the whole care chain. The assistant nurses were not educated to see the whole care system and needs of a patient. This setup was very expensive for society.

SW: What did you do after working as a community nurse?

GR: I worked as a care manager. In the Netherlands, there are many ways of describing managers in healthcare. I was a head nurse, team leader, and manager. All those words describe the managerial role. The organization I worked for had one hundred and fifty employees when I started. When I left after twenty-two years, the same organization had grown to twenty-three thousand people. All care organizations moved, merged, and became large entities. I think this growth was typical for that period in the Netherlands.

SW: Were these private organizations or public?

GR: Those were private, not for profit organizations paid for by the government.

SW: Did you work with Jos de Blok during that period?

GR: Yes. We worked together, but I was unaware of it at that time. Mr. de Blok worked at the psychiatric hospital twenty-five years ago. Afterward, he worked at a large home-care organization in the east of the Netherlands. This organization was different than the one I worked at, but the two organizations were often in contact and exchanging knowledge. We met each other a few times. In 2007, he founded Buurtzorg and asked me to come over and work as a nurse coach. This was an exciting offer, which I accepted.

SW: Who came up with the philosophy of nurse coaches?

GR: Mr. de Blok came up with his own model. In this model, self-organizing teams replace management. Mr. de Blok invented the role of nurse coaches. This important role supported and assisted the self-organizing teams. At the start of Buurtzorg, all of these teams had a nurse coach.

SW: What is the role of a nurse coach at Buurtzorg?

GR: The nurse coaches assist and support the teams. Nurse coaches advise the teams in their decision making processes. The role of a nurse coach depends on the needs of the team. If the team is new, the nurse coach plays a more active support role than for more mature teams. Many times the teams ask their nurse coach for advice.

SW: How many nurse coaches does Buurtzorg have today?

GR: Today around fifteen nurse coaches work at Buurtzorg. Every nurse coach handles a region in the Netherlands that contains around fifty teams. As a result, nurse coaches travel a lot. I started to work as a nurse coach in Amsterdam and the surrounding region.

SW: What are some of the most rewarding and hard parts of coaching?

GR: The rewarding part is that it is amazing to be able to visit the teams to see how they work. It is beautiful to see what the teams are doing and how they stay in contact with the patients and the whole network around the patients and to hear the patient view on the care process. The professionals in the teams are great at arranging the whole care process and taking care of their patients. They find solutions that I think managers and policymakers would never have found. At Buurtzorg, we give the freedom, the space, and the trust that the teams need. We do this without saying, "Well, you are on your own."

It is rewarding to be a part of the teams' care process and to help them to find their way. The best working style for one team might be different from that of another team. These differences are sometimes also what makes my job difficult. To work as a nurse coach limits your ability to help teams in their decision making process. You cannot decide for the teams. When I see the teams struggle, I want to help them. I want to make the right decision for them, but it is not up to me to decide. These situations are sometimes difficult.

I see Buurtzorg as a whole team, from the back office to the nurse coaches. As a team, we all try to support the self-organizing teams so that they can give the right care to their clients. As a result, the clients are able to live life as autonomously as possible.

SW: What are some of the characteristics that can help a nurse coach in his or her role?

GR: To be curious, friendly, and interested in people. It is also important to be able to look and listen to a team and to refocus on a care process without judging. The ability to stay in contact with and build up a relationship with the teams is also important. This team relationship is very important within Buurtzorg.

One of the first books that Mr. de Blok wrote about our model concerned building up relationships and then providing care. Before the teams care for a new client, they have a coffee together with the patient. Coffee is important in the Netherlands. Coffee is an important way to socialize and stay in contact with people. To drink coffee together builds trust in the team-client relationship. The coffee time shows the patients that we take time for them and that the team is there for them. The team and client have time to connect with each other. The teams build up relationships with their clients and families. This relationship building is the same as what a nurse coach is doing with his or her team.

SW: Do you train other nurse coaches?

GR: We train new nurse coaches on the job. We had two new colleagues in the last six months. We trained these new nurse coaches on the job. The new nurse coaches join the more experienced nurse coaches at work. We discuss different situations and how we help the new nurse coaches to find their own way. The best working style for one nurse coach might be different than that of another nurse coach. Just as I talked about before, when we help the teams find their own way. It is important to find your own way because, as a nurse coach, your work has to fit you. There is no one way that we work at Buurtzorg.

SW: Do you also receive training from external organizations?

GR: Yes. The organization we cooperate with is called the Institute for Cooperation Affairs. They train all of our teams and coaches at Buurtzorg.

SW: What kind of training does the institute offer?

GR: The Institute for Cooperation Affairs trains us on how to communicate, how to work together, how to work as a self-organizing team, and how to arrange and structure meetings. We use solution driven interaction methods. These methods are important when making decisions based on consensus. This is a process that the teams use to reach decisions. These decisions relate to the care that they give. The institute trains all teams and nurse coaches at Buurtzorg in this method.

SW: If you have a self-organizing team of six to twelve nurses and a nurse quits, who hires the new nurse?

GR: The team. It is also up to the team to decide how to design the recruitment and interview process. I used to be responsible for fifty-seven teams. I saw fifty-seven different ways of recruiting, planning, and arranging interviews. Some teams invite a potential nurse to come over for tea or lunch. Others invite them to join a nurse and visit the clients before their interview. The recruitment process has to fit with the team. The teams can also ask their nurse coach for advice or to join an interview session. The nurse coaches only advise and train their teams. The nurse coaches never decide on a new colleague for the team.

SW: Do you usually hire younger nurses or more experienced nurses?

GR: We prefer a mix, but we seldom have the luxury of hiring whomever we want. We often advise the teams to make a recruitment profile for a new team member. Team composition and experience is important to define before identifying a new profile.

SW: Do the nurses work alone at a patient home or do they work in pairs?

GR: Our nurses always work alone, except during special or complex occasions. The nurses feel like part of a team. The clients also say that a team is taking care of them.

SW: Does a nurse have access to an in-house doctor that he or she can consult over the telephone?

GR: Yes, but they are not in house doctors. In this neighborhood, for example, there is a team just around the corner. When the nurses start to work in a new neighborhood, they must first contact all of the general practitioners in the area. These nurses make sure to visit all the doctors by introducing themselves and explaining how Buurtzorg works. This introduction is very important, since the general practitioners often provide care for the clients. The nurses also give the doctors their phone numbers. The doctors can then call the nurse in case one of their patients needs homecare. Once the nurse is responsible for the homecare of a patient, the nurse contacts the general practitioner as needed.

SW: I think Buurtzorg has succeeded well in care coordination with doctors.

GR: Yes. What we see in Buurtzorg is that the nurses connect with the doctors when necessary. When the nurses visit their clients, they only call the doctor if it is urgent. The doctors know our nurses. The doctors know that the Buurtzorg nurses will only call them for important reasons.

SW: Do you share patient records with the general practitioners?

GR: Yes. We share information, but not electronically. We are still waiting to adopt digital information sharing.

SW: Is it the same for the emergency hospital? If one of your clients has an urgent visit to the hospital, do you know what is happening at the hospital? When the patient then returns back home, how does that communication work?

GR: Yesterday, for example, I had a meeting with a community nurse. She told me that the day before, she visited her clients. During her visit, she noticed that something was wrong with a patient. She ran all the tests on the patient and then called the doctor. The nurse and doctor talked and had a good discussion. The doctor then called the hospital to discuss the case with the doctor at the hospital. Five minutes later, the doctor phoned the nurse back and said that he had already sent an ambulance. The nurse then informed the patient and the family about the situation. The nurse also prepared all the necessary patient information. She called the pharmacist and asked for the patient's list of medications. The patient then went to the hospital while the nurse kept in contact with the family. The next day, the nurse visited the hospital to exchange information with the hospital staff. The nurse kept the family informed. She also stayed in contact with the hospital because the client would soon come home again and shift to her responsibility.

I think this coordination is a key strength of Buurtzorg. This strength turns into a weakness in many other care systems that we looked at. It is wrong to say that hospital care is the responsibility of the hospital and homecare is our responsibility. It is also important that the nurses feel the freedom to maintain contact. In other organizations, the nurses know that this contact is important. However, they are dependent on a set budget. The budget limits the nurses. They are only able to do things that are chargeable. You are not allowed to visit the hospital to exchange information or to gather information about a potential client.

A hospital might call the nurse regarding a potential client who goes home needing care. At Buurtzorg, the nurses visit the client at the hospital if it is necessary to meet with them and the family. The nurses can then prepare what is needed before the patient goes home. This process keeps the family relaxed when the patient comes home. The preparations also give the nurse a good picture of the client's needs. The nurses have time to explore the whole situation, to know what is needed, and to prepare this once the client comes home. Nurses in other organizations can only make these preparations after the patient responsibility has shifted from the hospital to the homecare organization.

SW: You work with neighbors, family members, and other people who are close to the individuals at home. You call this the person's network. The nurses know the neighborhood. What are examples of the resources that you unlock around the person at home?

GR: At Buurtzorg, we work on self-management for all our clients. We also look at neighborhood resources. We empower our clients. We believe that autonomy is important. We are not there to take over and paralyze the regular routines of the client and her family. From the beginning of our engagement with a new client, it is clear for us how we will work. If the client's children are away, we call the children and ask the client to invite one of them to our next visit. It is important for the children to visit their parent at home to see what they can do and to understand how they are involved. We then explain to the children what we are doing, what we will be doing, and how we would like to stay in contact with them. It is important to build a relationship with the family during those first weeks. At Buurtzorg, we take time and effort to get to know the client, which people are important in his or her life, and who might be supportive.

271

SW: Do you talk to neighbors?

GR: Yes, if necessary. We ask the client for permission first. We ask if they are close with their neighbors, with someone at church, or with people from a club. Sometimes the nurse also looks around the neighborhood for someone who can provide care. The nurses must be creative. The longer a team handles a neighborhood, the more they build up this network of neighborhood care. The team knows how their clients live and who cooks for them every week. One person might cook some extra food and bring it over to the client or even drive the client to the hospital. This is how the team maintains contact in an organic way.

SW: At a patient home, the assistant nurse might shower the patient, while the nurse looks at a bed sore. A physical therapist might train the muscles of the patient, while a dementia nurse cares for her medications. Do the nurses at Buurtzorg do all that?

GR: Yes. Our nurses do most of it, but they are not physical therapists. I think it works differently in the Netherlands than in other countries, where nurses are also trained in physical therapy. At Buurtzorg, nurses are not trained in physical therapy. Instead, all of our nurses are generalists. In fact, everyone who works for Buurtzorg is a generalist. In our teams, there will always be someone responsible for the morning visit and showering as well as tending the wound. There might also be someone in the team more trained or more experienced in dementia, for example. This person might then be the one responsible for a client with dementia. This responsibility does not prevent the other nurses from visiting the client with dementia. Instead, the responsible nurse might be the one to train colleagues regarding the situation.

SW: Is it always the same nurse that visits a client?

GR: No. The only exception might be if a client needs advice once a week or once every two weeks. However, most of our clients need more regular care. For visits three times a week, every day, or twice a day, different nurses will come to the client's home. The number of different nurses corresponds to the size of the team, which is, at most, twelve people. The maximum number is usually around seven for clients that need care twice a day.

SW: If the nurses do all these different tasks, they must be humble. Have they ever refused to do a specific task, like shower a patient?

GR: I do not think it is humility. We see it as part of nursing. To shower a client is equally important as a complex technique. The nurses are aware of this, so for me it is not about humility.

SW: Is that attitude something you see all over your country? Do nurses with that attitude exist all over the Netherlands or is it unique to Buurtzorg?

GR: I think it is a fundamental attitude of every nurse. However, this attitude has disappeared throughout the years. Today, the whole care system with its organizations direct the bachelor nurses and district nurses to a position in which they only perform technical tasks. The organizations view these nurses as too highly educated and expensive to do the more simple tasks. These nurses end up at the office. It is important to take a holistic approach. At Buurtzorg, we look at the whole client and the client's well-being. I think it helps the nurses to go back to the fundamental way of looking at their profession.

SW: Does the educational system contribute to the prevalent attitude?

GR: Maybe. It might be helpful if the educational system changed. Today, the bachelor of nursing education almost neglects the real fundamental care. Instead, nursing education is more about management and other things.

SW: You talk about the autonomy and the professionalism of the nurses. You also mentioned the continuity of care, with only seven people visiting a patient. This fundamental care increases the quality of care, but it also impacts costs. At Buurtzorg, you managed to lower or at least maintain the costs. How is that?

GR: What we have seen is that we are less expensive. We are less expensive because we take time to build relationships. It takes time to build up a relationship in the beginning of a client's care process. We spend more time, but we also save more money in this client situation. As a result, we know how to work on self-management for the client. We also know how to reduce time and costs, and how to keep the care level low. That is an important factor to lower the costs.

We also have small teams of highly educated nurses. These nurses work together and keep each other updated. These small teams prevent unnecessary client visits. In other organizations and teams, unnecessary client visits happen quite often. These teams rarely contact each other to exchange information. The teams detach their own nurses from situations and keep them uninformed. The nurses become strangers to their own clients. The nurses only receive their schedule for the evening and make sure to do their own tasks. If their task is to change the bandage, they do the task without looking at the wound.

In these teams, there is no communication, no interaction, and no helping each other. In the long run, this way of working is more expensive than the way we are able to work now at Buurtzorg. We are well informed and know each other. At Buurtzorg, we know that our nurses react if they see something is wrong with the client. In the example I gave earlier, as the nurse entered the house she noticed there was something wrong with the client. This nurse knew her client and reacted appropriately to the situation.

Our small teams also lead to fewer unplanned readmissions, which makes the Buurtzorg model less expensive. Our more highly educated nurses know what is going on in their teams. This information helps them to contact the general practitioner at an earlier stage. If the nurses note that something is wrong with the patient, they can intervene and see what is needed. The nurses can then ask a general practitioner to come over or do whatever is needed. If they instead wait to intervene, the client will most likely turn into an unplanned readmission.

SW: Can you tell us about your upcoming work as an international coordinator for Buurtzorg?

GR: Yes. About one year ago, Mr. de Blok asked me to think about joining as international coordinator at Buurtzorg. I was a nurse coach from Amsterdam that liked to host international guests. My job helped the international arm of Buurtzorg to grow organically. People from abroad stayed in Amsterdam and wanted to visit Buurtzorg. As a nurse coach responsible for this area, I enjoyed hosting international visitors and telling them about Buurtzorg. That is how I grew into the position as an international coordinator. I combined my role as nurse coach and international coordinator. I recently decided to go full time with the international arm of Buurtzorg. This was a big decision for me. As a nurse coach, I love to meet the teams, to be together with them, and to hear about their experience and processes. On the other hand, globalization is moving so fast that it is amazing. I want to be part of that global move. I am happy about my decision to go full time in international work.

It is Mr. de Blok who is on the frontline of our international work. International organizations and governments invite Mr. de Blok as a speaker to explain why and how he started Buurtzorg. He is a visionary who enjoys traveling.

He works on the frontline of Buurtzorg. Once he spreads the philosophy of Buurtzorg, I step in to coordinate and follow up, as much as possible. I can see that we are entering a new stage. We have invested for years. We worked hard to explain who we are, what we did, and what we are still doing. Now, we must take a concrete step. Some countries want to start projects or have already started projects with Buurtzorg. We must think about building up social platforms, franchising, joint ventures, and trainings. We had to create a training program for these new projects. This next step for Buurtzorg is exciting. It will be interesting to meet new people from other cultures and see how we can help each other without copying too much. I think it will work.

SW: Was the strategy of Buurtzorg to expand internationally from the start?

GR: No. People wanted us to expand. I think that is how Buurtzorg works. We do not have global strategies or structured plans for the next five years. I think our future will come naturally. All the interest from abroad surprised us. Buurtzorg grew through the many publications and writings about our model and philosophy.

SW: Please talk a little bit about your global expansion. Where is Buurtzorg present right now?

GR: We have invested in the United States, where we work with a small team in the city of Stillwater, Minnesota. We also have two teams in Sweden. A Swedish couple that used to live in the Netherlands started the two Swedish teams under the name Grannvård. The wife used to work with Buurtzorg in the Netherlands. She had an idea and asked us if she could start a team in Sweden. That is a great example of how we work. People feel the freedom to contribute new ideas and to see how it works. That is how Grannvård started in Sweden.

SW: Did Buurtzorg also invest in Grannvård? What other investments have you made?

GR: Yes, Buurtzorg invested in Grannvård, but I see Grannvård as the investment of the founders. The wife invested her time. To start two teams in another country requires twenty-four hours, seven days a week.

We also invested in Japan. That is another example of a successful information exchange between a Japanese professor, Satoko Hotta, and Mr. de Blok. After a few years working with a Japanese organization, we started the Orange Cross Foundation in Tokyo. We ran this project for a year. Forty-five organizations signed up for the project. Every organization worked on a transition plan. We tried to help by going through the transition plan and providing training on how our model works. Last night, I got an email from one of the team members in this project. He was very proud to announce the launch of his first Buurtzorg team in Japan. This is great news.

SW: How many teams are there in Japan now?

GR: This was the first team to start. We have forty-five organizations on the project. The next step is for the organizations to ask for a license at the Orange Cross Foundation. Then we will continue to train and advise them. Last week, we had a group of thirty people visiting us at Buurtzorg for a week of training about our model and experience.

SW: Where do you have that training? What type of training do you offer?

GR: This time, our Japanese visitors stayed in a small Dutch city for a week. We created a training program for their visit.

The aim of the program was to share the experience and practice the daily work of Buurtzorg. We have many teams in the host city. The program also included three days of joint team activities. The care group from Japan received more practical training since they were more informed than other guests. After the first few days of joint team activities, the group from Japan understood our concept. They understood the client center, the freedom for our nurses, the trust in our teams, and the relationship building.

SW: How does the training in practical experience work? Do you have someone in Japan who trains them as well?

GR: Yes. The Japanese professor, Ms. Hotta, is adapting the Buurtzorg model to the Japanese context. She does a great job and is important to the whole project.

SW: How do you think she bridges your model? What are the critical elements of the model that she translates into the Japanese context?

GR: She is well informed about the whole Buurtzorg model. Sometimes, when Mr. de Blok and I hear her talk, we say she knows better than us about how the model works. That is important. She is also a clever lady. She is knowledgeable about the Japanese context and healthcare system. In Japan, she is a leader on aging. She can translate our model into their situation. This bridge helps the healthcare organizations to apply the Buurtzorg theory with its fundamentals in Japan.

SW: Do you work in any other countries in Asia?

GR: Yes. We are exploring opportunities in Singapore and South Korea. We are close to receiving a grant in South Korea. We are in contact with both the government and organizations interested in starting teams with us. In China, we have a small first team located in Shanghai.

SW: Does Mr. de Blok travel much?

GR: Yes. He travels in Asia and through Europe. He travels around to network. Mr. de Blok does an amazing job. He is great at building up a network. He looks for the right people to collaborate with in the various countries. The network helps him find models to start up.

SW: Are you the person who maintains contact with everyone in the Netherlands?

GR: Yes. I work in collaboration with Mr. de Blok. I follow up his work and help him with what he needs. I also prepare the training sessions we talked about. I am the one who keeps in contact with everyone. I also think about potential contacts for Buurtzorg. That is my role for now. The international arm is new for us. We are exploring my role step by step to see what is needed. We do this in close contact with Mr. de Blok. It is important to know what he thinks is right, where he wants to go, and what he needs help with.

SW: Thank you so much, Gertje, for sharing your experiences at Buurtzorg.

GR: Thank you.

— END OF INTERVIEW —

Supporting the Caregiver

An interview with **Mary Mittelman**

Background

The NYU Caregiver Intervention is an evidence based program that provides support to spouses, partners, and families who are caring for a relative with dementia. Dr. Mary Mittelman and the expert clinicians in her NYU School of Medicine laboratory developed and tested the intervention for nearly thirty years. In the past decade, there have been many community translations of the NYU Caregiver Intervention. To meet the demand for trained counselors, Dr. Mittelman and her team have created an online training course for social workers and other social service clinicians to become certified in the intervention so they can bring it to their organizations or communities. The basic training is a ten-hour course. If the learner watches all of the case studies in full, the course takes twenty-four hours.

Research on the intervention began in 1987 when the National Institutes of Health funded a randomized controlled trial. The researchers found the caregivers in the treatment group experienced fewer symptoms of depression, were more satisfied with the support they received from family and friends, were less reactive to the behavior of the person with dementia, and were physically healthier than those in the control group who received the usual care provided in the laboratory at NYU. These changes enabled the caregivers to keep their spouse or partner with dementia at home with them for an average of a year and a half longer than those in the control group. They also coped better when their loved one moved into a nursing home or passed away.

During the research period, counselors responded to caregivers in the control group when they asked for assistance. However, those in the control group did not receive the six individual and family counseling sessions that participants in the treatment group received. The researchers concluded that mobilizing family support is the single most important factor in caregiver well-being.

Most often caregivers wish to keep their older relative with dementia at home as long as possible.

The components of the intervention include individual and family counseling, recommendation of support group participation, and ad hoc counseling as needed. The individual and family counseling sessions occur within four to six months of a comprehensive intake evaluation. Counselors offer support throughout the entire course of the caregiving process and up to two years after the death of the person with dementia. The counseling has elements of coaching and sometimes mediation with the caregiver's family. The counseling is individualized to the caregivers' needs and desires. Most of the time, these desires include being able to keep their family members with dementia at home, rather than putting them into a residential care facility.

Caregivers, particularly if they are the spouses or partners of the person with dementia, often become isolated from family and friends. They may avoid the company of others because of the stigma associated with the illness. They may also not know how to ask or what is reasonable to ask of family and friends. Even well meaning family members may not know how to interact with the primary caregiver in a constructive and supportive manner. Caregivers often wait to seek help until they or their relatives with dementia are in crisis. They are regularly put in the position of making choices without sufficient knowledge about dementia and the best care options for the person with the illness or themselves.

The individual and family counseling sessions in the NYU Caregiver Intervention focus on improving social support for the caregiver by enhancing the positive aspects and reducing the negative aspects of family interactions. The intervention provides education as needed about the causes and possible responses to the symptoms of dementia that the caregiver's relative may experience as the disease progresses. Counselors help the caregiver and family members to develop a plan for sharing the care now and in the future. During the study period, the intervention was provided with federal grant funding and was free to caregivers.

In the fall of 2015, New York State Governor Andrew M. Cuomo awarded a five-year, seven-and-a-half-million-dollar grant to NYU Langone Medical Center to launch the Family Support Program. The program provides support, counseling, and referrals to community resources for those in New York City who are caring for a relative with Alzheimer's disease and related dementias. The funding for ten such programs throughout New York State is at least in part due to the research and proven outcomes that provided an evidence base for the effectiveness of counseling and support interventions like the intervention developed by Dr. Mittelman and her team.

"This grant provides a unique opportunity to enact a model of the best possible care and support services for those caring for people with Alzheimer's disease," says Dr. Mittelman. "These caregivers face an incredible burden to their own mental and physical health as they provide care for their relatives affected with dementia."

The outcomes of the studies of the NYU Caregiver Intervention have been widely published in peer reviewed journals. In the past decade, there have been many government supported translations of the intervention by communities in the United States, as well as new randomized controlled trials. The article "Translating Research into Practice: Case Study of a Community-Based Dementia Caregiver Intervention" details the challenges and outcomes of the implementation of the NYU Caregiver Intervention at fourteen sites in Minnesota.

A report by Act on Alzheimer's describes a research model that estimated the economic impact on the state of Minnesota if at-home caregivers for those with dementia participated in the NYU Caregiver Intervention. Among other projections, the researchers estimated that if thirty percent of the caregivers were to participate in the intervention, the state would save as much as one and one-quarter of a billion dollars in direct healthcare costs between 2010 and 2025.

A report by the University of Pittsburgh Health Policy Institute calls for evidence based policy change at the state and federal levels to support family caregivers. The report acknowledges the benefit of caregiver support and suggests that there are not enough such programs to meet the expanding need.

Dr. Mittelman also founded The Unforgettables Chorus. The New York City-based chorus is made up of people with dementia and their family members and friends. The chorus gives members the chance to get out and enjoy learning to sing and perform together. It also serves as social support for the caregivers. As they rehearse and perform regularly for the community, caregivers are able to interact with others like themselves in a normal environment. The chorus has been featured in publications including the *Huffington Post*, the *New York Daily News*, and the *National Herald* (an online Greek newspaper). It has also been broadcast by news programs on ABC and PBS. Dr. Mittelman hopes to expand the number of choruses like the Unforgettables. She also plans to conduct a rigorous study of its benefits to both the participants with dementia and their caregivers.

In this interview, Dr. Mittelman discusses the NYU Caregiver Intervention from its inception to how it has evolved over nearly thirty years. She also details her plans for additional innovative caregiver interventions.

About Mary Mittelman

Mary S. Mittelman is a Research Professor in the Department of Psychiatry at the New York University School of Medicine. She is an epidemiologist who has been developing and evaluating psychosocial interventions for people with cognitive impairment and their family members for more than three decades. For more than twenty years, she was Principal Investigator of the National Institutes of Health-funded study of the NYU Caregiver Intervention. The results of the intervention have been published widely.

Dr. Mittelman has won many awards including the first global award for psychosocial research in Alzheimer's and dementia. The NYU Caregiver Intervention was named "the best evidence based intervention for people with dementia and their carers." The award was granted by the Alzheimer's Disease International and Fondation Médéric Alzheimer. Dr. Mittelman and her colleagues have developed online training for social service professionals as well as a telehealth version of the NYU Caregiver Intervention.

In the past decade, Dr. Mittelman has also been evaluating and developing interventions that include the person with dementia together with the caregiver. She is the founder of a chorus for people with dementia and their family members called The Unforgettables. The chorus rehearses and gives regular concerts at Saint Peter's Church in Manhattan.

INTERVIEW

Jean Galiana (JG): What inspired you to start the New York University Caregiver Intervention?

Mary Mittelman (MM): My initial motivation, as well as the motivation of most of the people I know who are involved in family caregiver work, is that we had a relative or friend with dementia. And it is likely that many of us will also have dementia one day.

I am a psychiatric epidemiologist by training. I drafted a grant proposal to study families. I sent it to Steven Ferris who was the head of what has now become the Alzheimer's Disease Center here at NYU. He introduced me to four women who had developed strategies to help family caregivers. They were talking to and helping the caregivers while the people with dementia were being evaluated. I said to these four women, "What do these people all have in common?" They said, "Nothing." I said, "Well, I am an epidemiologist. I want to draft a grant proposal to test whether what you have been doing is effective." I needed a theme. "What do they have in common?" They insisted that there is not a specific theme that caregivers have in common. I decided that they knew more than I did and that the theme should be "every caregiver is different." This meant that, to be effective, an intervention has to be individualized to each caregiver's strengths, weaknesses, and needs.

I formalized and created a structure for the caregiver intervention that the clinicians at NYU had been providing and drafted a grant proposal in late 1985. It was funded to begin in August 1987. The National Institute of Mental Health originally supported it. The National Institute on Aging took over the funding in 1991. The proposal was to conduct a randomized control trial of caregiver counseling and support in a formalized way. We began with a comprehensive assessment to get a profile of the caregiver and of the person with dementia for whom he or she cared. In the initial study, all the caregivers were spouse or partner caregivers. Over a period of nine and a half years, we ended up enrolling four hundred and six caregivers. The first cohort was two hundred and six couples. I then received a second grant and enrolled two hundred more. I started out with a four year-grant and I ended up with over twenty years of funding sequentially.

We followed some of these caregivers for as long as eighteen years. We had less than a five percent dropout rate while the person with dementia was still at home, which is extraordinary in an older adult population. Most of the caregivers were also older adults since they were spouses or partners. I attribute the low dropout rate to the fact that even the control group received a lot of support. The intervention had some structured and some unstructured components. There was the evaluation. Then the caregivers were randomized. Those in the treatment group had six individual and family counseling sessions. It began with an individual session for the spouse or partner caregiver, four family sessions, and then another individual session followed.

JG: How many of the caregivers' family members participated?

MM: Two or more. We had as many as thirteen. We consider family to be anyone who the caregiver considers to be family. Caregivers are not necessarily relatives. Caregivers can be best friends, if they feel like family. We never had children under eighteen, but sometimes we had three generations in one room. Certain cultures had bigger families on average than others.

After the first individual session, there were four family sessions, and then there was another individual counseling session. Then we did a follow up assessment, at which time we urged the caregivers to join support groups. The counselors were available to the caregiver and the family any time they needed help. The counselor would hand out a card to every family member. At the beginning, ad hoc counseling was not explicitly defined as part of the formal counseling. We noticed people were calling the counselors when they needed additional advice, referrals, and support, and that they often commented on how important a resource this was. So we added it as a formal component of the NYU Caregiver Intervention, calling it "ad hoc counseling." Even if caregivers did not call, they would often say at the follow up, "I did not think I could cope and then I remembered I had your card. I was able to cope because I knew I could call you. The card is like a life preserver."

Because of the human nature of the program, there was no way we could stop people from getting help. The non-placebo control group would often call the counselors. When they came in with a person with dementia they often would seek out the counselors. The one component that they did not get was the family counseling. For that reason, we came to believe that the family involvement component was the potent part of the package.

The package as a whole is crucial. For example, you cannot provide family counseling alone, even though it is the most potent ingredient. A report in *PLOS ONE* details the efforts of one organization in the Netherlands that attempted to use the family component on its own, and to space the sessions over a one-year period. It did not work. The NYU Caregiver Intervention is a package and each part of the package has a contribution. It is like baking a cake. You cannot take an ingredient out and get the same cake. If you did, you would make a different cake.

Each part of the counseling was individualized and devoted to what the participants said they needed. The counselors always tried to make a point of helping the caregiver to understand the importance of involving their families. Before anything was ever published, there was one female caregiver who appeared on Eyewitness News with Emma Shulman and me. Emma, with whom I shared an office for about five years, worked with me until she was ninety-eight. She and I and the caregiver were all invited. During the interview, I overheard the caregiver say that she would never have survived without the counselor.

I remembered that the caregiver was in the control group. I was worried that, if she was so grateful, there would be no difference in outcome between the treatment and control groups. Then, a few months later, she placed her husband in a nursing home. We had questionnaires for everything. We asked her why she placed her husband in a nursing home. She said, "My sons never helped me." The one component she did not receive was the family counseling. So, do we know whether she asked for help and whether her sons would have helped her if she asked? There are any number of reasons why family counseling can improve the situation. In some families, the caregiver will say, "They ought to know enough to offer. I shouldn't need to ask." Other caregivers will say, "They have their own lives to lead. They should not be bothered. I am going to do this by myself." Other caregivers keep completely hidden.

Social support is the mediator of all the other outcomes that we found. Compared to the control group, which received much more than a placebo, the caregivers in the treatment group had fewer symptoms of depression. They had much less severe stress reactions to the patient's behavior despite the fact that the patient's behavior did not change. They had better self-rated health. These outcomes led to the ensuing outcome that the government loved. We postponed nursing home placement for a year and a half longer among people whose caregivers were in the treatment group than among those in the control group. Satisfaction with social support, with emotional support from family and friends, with assistance from family and friends, and the number of people to whom the primary caregiver felt close, made the difference. Those were the mediators of all the other outcomes.

Once I had demonstrated that the intervention was effective, I felt like, while it is not a university professor's job, it was my job to make it available as widely as possible. Most people who work in university life focus on getting tenure and promotions and more grants. I think I probably sacrificed some of that because I focused on making the intervention available.

The intervention was written about in peer reviewed journals. But those readers are not the people the intervention supports. Our challenge was to connect the intervention to the millions of people whom it could support.

The next development was that people started to implement the intervention in the way they thought it was supposed to be done but not the way we designed it. They were not getting the same results, because they were not doing it properly. That is when we knew we had to publish the intervention process in detail. So we wrote a book entitled *Counseling the Alzheimer's*

Caregiver: A Resource for Health Care Professionals, which was published by American Medical Association Press in 2003.

JG: It must be disappointing when you hear of other organizations doing only part of the intervention.

MM: Yes. One organization in the Netherlands decided they would just conduct the family part of the intervention. They conducted one family session every three months but measured outcomes after every four months. After one year, they had no positive outcomes to report. I finally said to the principal investigator of this grant, "If you were told to give your child penicillin every six hours and you thought you would space it out differently and give it to them once a day, do you think you would get the same outcome?" We were concerned that organizations would not do the intervention properly.

This is what spurred us to develop a formal online training course. We received a Small Business Innovation Research Grant from the National Institute on Aging to develop the detailed training. We created the training program with Healthcare Interactive. The training included specific and extensive videos of case studies as well as text and video commentary. Now any organization in the world can train their staff to do the New York University Caregiver Intervention properly and in its entirety.

We developed that training and then we did a cluster randomized control trial of the training. I reported at the Alzheimer's Association International Conference last year in Washington that the randomized control trial showed no difference in knowledge of the intervention and understanding of it between clinicians who received the training in person and those who received it through our online program. The online training has some value over the in person training that we were doing before because you can do it in the middle of the night or on the weekend. If you lose an employee you do not need me to return to train the replacement.

JG: Please describe the pilot program you conducted in Minnesota.

MM: In approximately 2007 or 2008, the Administration on Aging started to send out calls for states to apply for funding to conduct trials of evidence based interventions. Minnesota was the first to conduct a translation of the NYU Caregiver Intervention. You may have seen the *Health Affairs* article, "Translating Research into Practice: Case Study of a Community-Based Dementia Caregiver Intervention." They enrolled two hundred eighty caregivers. California, Georgia, Wisconsin, Florida, Virginia, and Nevada also received funding from the Administration on Aging to conduct what they call "community translations" of the NYU Caregiver Intervention.

In addition, the Rosalynn Carter Institute for Caregiving funded pilot studies in Vermont, Nevada, and at an agency that provides care for the homebound in New York City. We also conducted the Three Country Study in Australia, the United Kingdom, and the United States. The study demonstrated outcomes similar to the original study, significantly reducing caregiver depression.

I realized that there were many caregivers who could not access the intervention either because they live nowhere near an experienced counselor or because their families are spread widely. I am committed to making the principles of the intervention available to as many caregivers as possible. I started thinking about rural caregivers and the many other factors barring people from getting counseling in person. They might live in Staten Island or Brooklyn and may not be able to get here. They might not like driving at night but their children are only available at night. We started getting requests to include family who were living in different states. They wanted to participate by phone. I heard it a couple of times and I thought, "We should do this intervention using video conferencing."

We developed a videoconferencing version of the intervention. It is only different in the sense that people do not need to be in the same room to participate. We use Zoom, which I chose because several people with dementia were using it to make conference calls and thought, "If they can do it, we should use it." We will be able to reach many more caregivers with this technology.

We are now doing a randomized control trial to compare the online version of the intervention to counseling on the phone. I do not want to be selling it if it does not have an evidence base behind it. I just found out this morning we have twenty-eight caregivers enrolled in the randomized control trial. We are hoping to have a total of two hundred and forty by the end of the year. We have counselors in many states now that are enrolling caregivers.

JG: How many organizations have implemented the initiative already?

MM: I think there have been fourteen translations and new randomized controlled trials. We recently concluded a trial in Israel that has yielded similar results to the research at NYU. Those results are soon to be published. We are also working in Paris with Saint Joseph hospital. And we are hoping to implement the intervention elsewhere in France. To me, there is no limit.

JG: Is the intervention training available in languages other than English?

MM: The intervention training is only available in English. We simultaneously developed it for Australia with a small grant that the University of Queensland received. I was a consultant and my colleague had a subcontract. With that grant, we translated the words that were not Australian. For example, "caregiver" became "carer." The training is narrated by a native Australian.

A year after we started training people in Australia, we video-taped one of the counselors who had the most experience providing live counseling with an Australian family. We have all the sessions, the evaluation, and the individual and family counseling with an Australian family available in the online training. Families are different. Cultures are different. Expectations are different. And language is different. That is why we customized the training to be specific for Australia.

JG: Do you plan to bring the intervention to other countries as well?

MM: Yes. But I would also like the training to be culturally relevant. We should begin by offering the existing training and then translate it into the culture. We can accomplish this by training people who speak both English and the native language of the country. It is not a matter of simply translating the language. We would need to understand other culturally relevant issues for caregiving in each country.

JG: Have you advocated for policy change in order to get the intervention reimbursed by insurers?

MM: I think our reliance on drugs and what doctors traditionally do is not sufficient for chronic care and illnesses like those that cause dementia. As a culture, we do not value support programs like the New York University Caregiver Intervention. It is time that insurers understand the importance of treating the caregiver, especially in the absence of disease altering medications. Helping the caregiver can save a lot of money in physical and mental healthcare costs for the caregiver. We do not think about that as often as we should. We have also mentioned the cost savings realized for the person with dementia because, with the caregiver intervention, the person can remain at home for an average of a year and a half longer.

I met with the Centers for Medicare and Medicaid Services.

They recommended looking for an opportunity to have a managed care company conduct a pilot test so that we could prove that we are saving healthcare costs, not only for the person with dementia but for the caregivers among their insured.

We need to find the right connections and legislative backing. There is a letter circulating in the Senate about caregiver interventions now. The letter mentions the New York University Caregiver Intervention and one other. There is evidence behind both of them that makes a clear case for providing interventions for the benefit of the patient as well as the caregiver.

JG: Please describe the grant that NYU recently received from the state.

MM: That was an exciting grant for us. In the fall of 2015, New York State Governor Andrew M. Cuomo awarded a five-year, seven-and-a-half-million-dollar grant to NYU Langone Medical Center to launch the Family Support Program that provides support, counseling, and referrals to community resources for those caring for a relative with Alzheimer's disease and related dementias throughout New York City.

JG: Are you designing additional caregiver support interventions?

MM: We think that older adults with other chronic illnesses—like multiple sclerosis for example—could also benefit from this kind of intervention. One of my best friends died with multiple sclerosis. I think the family would have benefited from a similar family intervention. We have also submitted proposals to design and evaluate interventions based on the same paradigm for traumatic brain injury.

We have a couple of innovations that we are including in our new five-year New York State funded Family Support Program, in which we will be providing caregiver support in the five boroughs of New York City. Darby Morhardt at Northwestern

University developed the Buddy Program, where first-year medical students become the companions of people in the early stage of dementia. We plan to expand that model here so that students in all the schools at New York University will be buddied with people in the early stage of dementia. They have things to teach each other. This program will also provide respite for the caregiver while the student is with the person with dementia. The students and the people with dementia will have an invaluable experience. Someone from the engineering school asked me what an engineering student could get out of this experience. I replied, "The engineer might be designing products for older adults with impairments. Why not have an older adult to talk to so they have a better idea of what would work?"

We also plan to add a peer mentoring program, which has already been successful in other contexts. We are going to engage people who have long experience being a caregiver to mentor other caregivers. The mentors could have lost the person with dementia, or might just have time available. They may wish to share their experiences and what they learned about how to get the help they needed. The mentors may offer ideas to make the new caregiver feel more comfortable about talking about being a caregiver to their family and friends. If they do not talk about their situation, they can become isolated and overwhelmed. I have already asked two of the people who are in The Unforgettables chorus who have lost their partner with dementia. They both want to be peer mentors.

We will be looking to connect with and provide counseling and support for the caregivers who, either because of the stigma of the illness or for other reasons, are trying to keep the dementia diagnosis secret. Perhaps they do not want to acknowledge the diagnosis themselves. I want to find those caregivers, to help them reduce their stress and isolation. I want to make it